D1462063

Spinal Cord Injury

Rehabilitation Medicine Quick Reference

Ralph M. Buschbacher, MD

Series Editor

Professor, Department of Physical Medicine and Rehabilitation
Indiana University School of Medicine
Indianapolis, Indiana

▪ Spine

André Panagos

▪ Spinal Cord Injury

Thomas N. Bryce

Forthcoming Volumes in the Series

Traumatic Brain Injury

Musculoskeletal, Sports, and Occupational Medicine

Pediatrics

Neuromuscular/EMG

Prosthetics

Stroke

Spinal Cord Injury

Rehabilitation Medicine Quick Reference

Thomas N. Bryce, MD

Associate Professor
Department of Rehabilitation Medicine
Mount Sinai School of Medicine
New York, New York

Associate Editors

Naomi Betesh, DO
Chief Resident
Department of Rehabilitation Medicine
Mount Sinai School of Medicine
New York, New York

Kristjan T. Ragnarsson, MD
Lucy G. Moses Professor and Chairman
Department of Rehabilitation Medicine
Mount Sinai School of Medicine
New York, New York

Avniel Shetreat-Klein, MD, PhD
Instructor
Department of Rehabilitation Medicine
Mount Sinai School of Medicine
New York, New York

Adam B. Stein, MD
Chairman
Department of Physical Medicine and Rehabilitation
The North Shore-Long Island Jewish Health System
Great Neck, New York

demos
MEDICAL
New York

Acquisitions Editor: Beth Barry
Cover Design: Steven Pisano
Compositor: NewGen North America
Printer: Bang Printing
Visit our website at www.demosmedpub.com

Medicine is an ever-changing science. Research and clinical experience are continually
expanding our knowledge, in particular our understanding of proper treatment and drug
therapy. The authors, editors, and publisher have made every effort to ensure that all information in this book is in accordance with the state of knowledge at the time of production of
the book. Nevertheless, the authors, editors, and publisher are not responsible for errors or
omissions or for any consequences from application of the information in this book and make
no warranty, express or implied, with respect to the contents of the publication. Every reader
should examine carefully the package inserts accompanying each drug and should carefully
check whether the dosage schedules mentioned therein or the contraindications stated by the
manufacturer differ from the statements made in this book. Such examination is particularly
important with drugs that are either rarely used or have been newly released on the market.

Library of Congress Cataloging-in-Publication Data

Spinal cord injury / editor, Thomas N. Bryce ; associate editors, Naomi Betesh ... [et al.].
     p. ; cm.—(Rehabilitation medicine quick reference)
 Includes bibliographical references and index.
 ISBN 978-1-933864-47-1
 1. Spinal cord—Wounds and injuries—Handbooks, manuals, etc. I. Bryce, Thomas N.
II. Series: Rehabilitation medicine quick reference.
 [DNLM: 1. Spinal Cord Injuries—rehabilitation—Handbooks. WL 39 S757 2010]
 RD594.3.S6683 2010
 616.7′3—dc22   2009024708

Special discounts on bulk quantities of Demos Medical Publishing books are available to cor-
porations, professional associations, pharmaceutical companies, health care organizations,
and other qualifying groups. For details, please contact:

Special Sales Department
Demos Medical Publishing
11 West 42nd Street, 15th Floor
New York, NY 10036
Phone: 800-532-8663 or 212-683-0072
Fax: 212-941-7842
Email: rsantana@demosmedpub.com

Made in the United States of America

09 10 11 12   5 4 3 2 1

*To the staff and patients of the Mount Sinai
Medical Center Spinal Cord Injury Unit*

Contents

Conditions

Interventions

Outcomes

List of Acronyms

ADL   activity of daily living
AIS   ASIA impairment scale
ASIA   American Spinal Injury Association
CSF   cerebrospinal fluid
CT   computed tomography
CVD   cardiovascular disease
EEG   electroencephalography
EKG   electrocardiogram
EMG   electromyography
GI   gastrointestinal
LMN   lower motor neuron
MRI   magnetic resonance imaging
ROM   range of motion
SCI   spinal cord injury
UMN   upper motor neuron
UTI   urinary tract infection

Series Foreword

The Rehabilitation Medicine Quick Reference (RMQR) series is dedicated to the busy clinician. While we all strive to keep up with the latest medical knowledge, there are many times when things come up in our daily practices that we need to look up. Even more importantly . . . look up quickly.

Those aren't the times to do a complete literature search or to read a detailed chapter or review article. We just need to get a quick grasp of a topic that we may not see routinely, or just to refresh our memory. Sometimes a subject comes up that is outside our usual scope of practice, but that may still impact our care. It is for such moments that this series has been created.

Whether you need to quickly look up what a Tarlov cyst is, or you need to read about a neurorehabilitation complication or treatment, RMQR has you covered.

RMQR is designed to include the most common problems found in a busy practice, but also a lot of the less common ones as well.

I was extremely lucky to have been able to assemble an absolutely fantastic group of editors. They in turn have harnessed an excellent set of authors. So what we have in this series is, I hope and believe, a tremendous reference set to be used often in daily clinical practice. As series editor, I have of course been privy to these books before actual publication. I can tell you that I have already started to rely on them in my clinic—often. They have helped me become more efficient in practice.

Each chapter is organized into succinct facts, presented in a bullet point style. The chapters are set up in the same way throughout all of the volumes in the series, so once you get used to the format, it is incredibly easy to look things up.

And while the focus of the RMQR series is, of course, rehabilitation medicine, the clinical applications are much broader.

I hope that each reader grows to appreciate the Rehabilitation Medicine Quick Reference series as much as I have. I congratulate a fine group of editors and authors on creating readable and useful texts.

Ralph M. Buschbacher, MD

Having a spinal cord injury (SCI) can profoundly change a person's life as it can affect nearly all the body systems. It also affects the perception of that person by others. Clinicians who treat persons with SCI need to not only be able to treat the medical complications that can result, but also treat the whole person, helping those affected to return to a productive life integrated within society. This book was developed for all physicians and other health care professionals involved in the care of persons with SCI to provide knowledge to help facilitate this process.

The book addresses over one hundred varied topics related to SCI, ranging from psychological adjustment to treatment of vocal fold paralysis. It is organized into three sections, the first includes the medical and psychological conditions associated with SCI; the second includes common interventions; while the last outlines expected functional outcomes. I hope you find it useful.

Thomas N. Bryce, MD

Contributors

AnneMarie Abdulrauf, MA, CCC-SLP
Consultant
St. Louis, Missouri

Kenneth W. Altman, MD, PhD, FACS
Director
Grabscheid Voice Center
Associate Professor of Otolaryngology
Mount Sinai School of Medicine
New York, New York

Gina Armstrong, MD
Resident
Department of Rehabilitation Medicine
Mount Sinai School of Medicine
New York, New York

Anousheh Behnegar, MD
Assistant Professor
Department of Rehabilitation Medicine
Mount Sinai School of Medicine
New York, New York

Liron Bensimon, DPT, CSCS
Advanced Clinician
Spinal Cord Injury Unit
Department of Rehabilitation Medicine
The Mount Sinai Medical Center
New York, New York

Naomi Betesh, DO
Chief Resident
Department of Rehabilitation Medicine
Mount Sinai School of Medicine
New York, New York

Thomas N. Bryce, MD
Associate Professor
Department of Rehabilitation Medicine
Mount Sinai School of Medicine
New York, New York

Stephen Burns, MD
Staff Physician
SCI Service
VA Puget Sound Health Care System
Associate Professor
Department of Rehabilitation Medicine
University of Washington
Seattle, Washington

Tanvir F. Choudhri, MD
Co-Director
Neurosurgical Spine Program
Assistant Professor of Neurosurgery
Department of Neurosurgery
Mount Sinai School of Medicine
New York, New York

Dana Spivack David, MS, CCC-SLP
Chief Speech Language Pathologist
Department of Rehabilitation Medicine
The Mount Sinai Medical Center
New York, New York

Kemesha L. Delisser, MD
Resident
Department of Rehabilitation Medicine
Mount Sinai School of Medicine
New York, New York

Richard Freiden, MD
Assistant Professor
Department of Rehabilitation Medicine
Mount Sinai School of Medicine
New York, New York

Sylvia G. Geraci, DO
Resident
Department of Physical Medicine and Rehabilitation
The North Shore-Long Island Jewish Health System
Great Neck, New York

Justin T. Hata, MD
Assistant Clinical Professor
Departments of Anesthesiology and Physical Medicine
and Rehabilitation
University of California School of Medicine, Irvine
Orange, California

Neil N. Jasey, Jr., MD
Instructor
Department of Rehabilitation Medicine
Mount Sinai School of Medicine
New York, New York

Youssef Josephson, DO
Resident
Department of Physical Medicine and Rehabilitation
The North Shore-Long Island Jewish Health System
Great Neck, New York

Jenny Lieberman, MSOTR/L, ATP
Advanced Clinical Specialist
Wheelchair Seating and Positioning
Department of Rehabilitation Medicine
The Mount Sinai Medical Center
New York, New York

Jung-Woo Ma, MD
Resident
Department of Rehabilitation Medicine
Mount Sinai School of Medicine
New York, New York

Donald SF Macron, MD, MA
Resident
Department of Rehabilitation Medicine
Mount Sinai School of Medicine
New York, New York

Melvin S. Mejia, MD
Assistant Professor
Department of Physical Medicine and Rehabilitation
Case Western Reserve University School of Medicine
MetroHealth Rehabilitation Institute of Ohio
Cleveland, Ohio

Greg Nemunaitis, MD
Associate Professor of Physical Medicine and
  Rehabilitation
Case Western Reserve University School of Medicine
Director of Spinal Cord Injury Rehabilitation
MetroHealth Rehabilitation Institute of Ohio
Cleveland, Ohio

Danielle Perret, MD
Director of Education
Division of Pain Medicine
Department of Anesthesiology and Perioperative Care
University of California School of Medicine, Irvine
Orange, California

Kristjan T. Ragnarsson, MD
Dr. Lucy G. Moses Professor
Chairman
Department of Rehabilitation Medicine
Mount Sinai School of Medicine
New York, New York

Igor Rakovchik, DO
Spinal Cord Injury Fellow
Department of Rehabilitation Medicine
Mount Sinai School of Medicine
New York, New York

Angela Riccobono, PhD
Senior Psychologist
Department of Rehabilitation Medicine
The Mount Sinai Medical Center
New York, New York

Kimberly Sackheim, DO
Resident
Department of Rehabilitation Medicine
Mount Sinai School of Medicine
New York, New York

Matthew M. Shatzer, DO
Residency Program Director
Chief of Physical Medicine and Rehabilitation
North Shore University Hospital
Great Neck, New York

Avniel Shetreat-Klein, MD, PhD
Instructor
Department of Rehabilitation Medicine
Mount Sinai School of Medicine
New York, New York

Harshpal Singh, MD
Resident
Department of Neurosurgery
Mount Sinai School of Medicine
New York, New York

Adam B. Stein, MD
Chairman
Department of Physical Medicine and Rehabilitation
The North Shore-Long Island Jewish Health System
Great Neck, New York

Chih-Kwang Sung, MD, MS
Laryngology Fellow
Department of Otolaryngology
Massachusetts Eye and Ear Infirmary
Harvard Medical School
Boston, Massachusetts

Melin Tan-Geller, MD
Laryngology Fellow
Mount Sinai School of Medicine
New York, New York

Jonathan M. Vapnek, MD
Clinical Associate Professor
Department of Urology
Mount Sinai School of Medicine
New York, New York

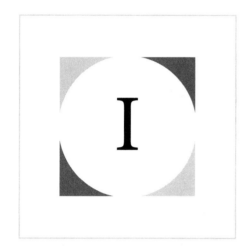

Conditions

Airway Issues: Tracheal Stenosis

Kenneth W. Altman MD PhD ■ Chih-Kwang Sung MD MS

Description

Tracheal stenosis is an abnormal narrowing of the tracheal lumen due to an intrinsic or extrinsic mass.

Etiology/Types

Etiology
- Intubation trauma
- Tracheostomy
- Neoplasm
- Infection
- External trauma
- Gastroesophageal reflux disease (GERD)
- Inflammatory/granulomatous/autoimmune disease
- Idiopathic

Types
- Congenital
- Acquired iatrogenic injuries are the most common cause
- Tracheostomy-related stenosis can be classified according to site of lesion: suprastomal, stomal, cuff, and cannula tip stenosis
- Cotton staging system: grade 1, <50% obstruction; grade 2, 50% to 70% obstruction; grade 3, 71% to 99% obstruction; and grade 4, complete obstruction

Epidemiology
- Incidence of postintubation or post-tracheostomy stenosis 10% to 22%, depending on duration and nature of intubation
- 1% to 2% are symptomatic or have severe stenosis

Pathogenesis

Acquired due to intubation tube cuff
- Excessive endotracheal (ET) tube or tracheostomy tube cuff pressure (>30 mm Hg) impairs mucosal capillary perfusion.
- Mucosal ischemia leads to ulcerations and chondritis.
- Lesions heal by fibrosis, resulting in progressive cicatricial stenosis.

Acquired due to tracheostomy tube
- Poor surgical technique or poor visualization/palpation of landmarks
- Traumatic crush injury during procedure inverting cricoid cartilage or tracheal rings into airway
- Trauma of posterior tracheal wall during dilation and tube insertion
- Stomal stenosis secondary to bacterial infection and chondritis, which precipitate inflammation and granulation
- Distal tracheal stenosis from tracheostomy tube tip irritation or aggressive suction trauma
- Granulation tissue can progress and heal by fibrosis

Risk Factors
- Prolonged intubation
- Type and size of ET tube
- Stomal infection
- Hypotension
- Tight fitting tracheal cannula
- Excessive tube motion
- Corticosteroids
- High tracheostomy
- Cricothyrotomy (cricothyroidotomy)
- Excessive resection of anterior tracheal ring or poor tracheostomy procedure technique

Clinical Features
- Cough
- Inability to clear secretions
- Exertional dyspnea
- Stridor (usually biphasic)
- Inability to tolerate capping of tracheostomy tube
- Aphonia

Natural History
- Prior history of neck trauma, intubation, or tracheostomy; symptoms may present within days.
- Symptoms may have sudden or gradual onset,
- Stenosis due to chronic inflammatory conditions or GERD is more likely to progress.
- Often asymptomatic until stenosis is >50% to 75% of lumen or diameter is <5 mm.

Diagnosis

Differential diagnosis
- Asthma
- Infection: supraglottitis, croup, bronchitis

History
- Trauma, intubation, or tracheostomy: days or weeks before onset of symptoms
- Dyspnea, increased work of breathing
- Aggravating factors: exercise, infection
- Recurrent pneumonia

Testing
- Helical computed tomography (CT) scan of neck and chest with fine cuts through the larynx and proximal trachea—preferred study
- Magnetic resonance imaging (MRI) to characterize soft tissue mass if present
- Pulmonary function testing (PFT)—may reveal fixed extrathoracic obstruction
- Flexible laryngoscopy
- Flexible or rigid bronchoscopy
- Direct microlaryngoscopy

Pitfalls
- Symptoms of asthma or wheezing may be confused with laryngotracheal stenosis.
- Asthma can be excluded based on PFT and successful response to treatment.

Red Flags
- Acute respiratory distress: requires securing of airway with tracheostomy or rigid bronchoscopy

Treatment

Medical
- Preventive measures: early tracheostomy; properly sized tubes; high volume, low-pressure cuffs
- Humidified air or oxygen
- Heliox therapy to temporarily reduce airway resistance
- Treatment of underlying medical causes of stenosis (eg, infectious or inflammatory)
- Antireflux management: dietary and lifestyle modifications, proton pump inhibitors, H2 blockers

Exercises
- General cardiovascular training to improve pulmonary requirements

Surgical
- Long-term tracheostomy
- Endoscopic repair: laser incision or excision, dilation
- Open repair: segmental tracheal resection with end-to-end anastomosis, laryngotracheoplasty with anterior or anterior-posterior cricoid split, and T-tube placement
- Stent placement

Consults
- Otolaryngology
- Cardiothoracic surgery

Complications of treatment
- Restenosis
- Migration or infection of stent
- Granulation tissue
- Mortality after end-to-end anastomosis up to 5% due to anastomosis breakdown and/or mediastinitis

Prognosis
- One-third of patients can be managed by laser excision, bronchoscopic dilation, or tracheal stenting.
- Two-thirds require open procedures.

Helpful Hints
- The goal of treatment is to improve airway function while retaining laryngeal function. Airway safety is paramount in all cases.

Suggested Readings
Epstein SK. Late complications of tracheostomy. *Resp Care.* 2005;50(4):542–549.

Sue RD, Susanto I. Long-term complications of artificial airways. *Clin Chest Med.* 2003;24(3):457–471.

Zias N, Chroneou A, Tabba MK, et al. Post tracheostomy and post intubation tracheal stenosis: Report of 31 cases and review of the literature. *BMC Pulm Med.* 2008;8:18.

Section I: Conditions

Airway Issues: Vocal Fold Paralysis

Kenneth W. Altman MD PhD ■ Melin Tan-Geller MD

Description

Vocal fold paralysis after spinal cord injury (SCI) is most commonly due to injury to the recurrent laryngeal nerve (RLN) and often leads to a weak or absent voice and can lead to aspiration.

Etiology/Types

- Congenital
- Traumatic
- Postsurgical
- Neoplastic
- Neuromuscular
- Infectious
- Vascular
- Idiopathic

Epidemiology

- Postsurgical paralysis occurs in approximately 2% to 6% of anterior cervical spine surgeries.
- True paralysis due to endotracheal intubation is rare and likely related to hyperinflation of the cuff.
- Paralysis due to brain stem stroke can occur but is rare.

Pathogenesis

- RLN injury is the most common cause of vocal fold immobility causing true paralysis or paresis.
- Superior laryngeal nerve injury can cause paresis.
- Immobility can occur from scarring, ankylosis, or dislocation of the arytenoids.
- A mass or neoplasm can limit vocal fold movement.

Risk Factors

- Surgery in proximity to RLN
- Endotracheal intubation

Clinical Features

- Unilateral paralysis: weak or breathy voice, change in pitch, weak cough and poor pulmonary secretion management, cough with eating or drinking, aspiration, choking
- Bilateral paralysis: stridor and airway obstruction if adducted position; aphonia and aspiration if abducted position

Natural History

- Postsurgical neuropraxia of the RLN has about a 30% to 50% likelihood of meaningful recovery by 6 months.
- Injuries due to intubation have about a 50% likelihood of recovery at 6 months.
- Complete nerve transactions are unlikely to recover.
- Without treatment, aspiration is the greatest risk.

Diagnosis

Differential diagnosis

- Vocal fold paresis
- Arytenoid dislocation/subluxation or fixation
- Laryngeal scar, web
- Posterior glottic stenosis
- Mass or neoplasm
- Degenerative neuromuscular disorder

History

- Neck or chest surgery
- Prolonged intubation
- Trauma to the neck
- Aspiration
- Choking
- Weak, breathy, or absent voice
- Change in pitch of voice
- Weak cough
- Cough with eating or drinking

Exam

- Asymmetric movement of the vocal folds
- Vocal fold bowing
- Tilting of the posterior larynx
- Incompetent closure of vocal folds on phonation
- Stridor on auscultation
- Aphonia

Testing

- Laryngeal electromyography (EMG) confirms impaired muscular recruitment, and determines presence of polyphasic potentials (reinnervation) or spontaneous activity (dennervation).
- Aspiration risk should be assessed with bedside swallow evaluation, flexible endoscopic evaluation of swallowing, or modified Barium swallow.

- An unexplained new-onset vocal paralysis should be assessed with CT neck/fine cuts of larynx with intravenous contrast to evaluate the course of the RLN.

Pitfalls
- Vocal fold immobility due to scar, stenosis, arytenoid dislocation, or ankylosis

Treatment

Medical
- Treatment is focused on improvement of voice quality if aspiration not present.

Exercises
- Voice therapy can offer patients useful compensatory exercises that improve voice quality and improve aspiration protection.

Surgical (for unilateral paralysis)
- Medialization for unilateral paralysis is performed either by injection of material into the vocal fold or with an implant augmenting the vocal fold.
- Reinnervation to the ansa cervicalis, phrenic nerve, preganglionic sympathetic neurons, hypoglossal nerve, and nerve-muscle pedicles are also employed.

Surgical (for bilateral paralysis)
- Tracheotomy may be required if airway patency is jeopardized by adducted bilateral vocal paralysis
- Cordotomy and arytenoidectomy with or without suture lateralization of the vocal fold for bilateral vocal paralysis.

- Unilateral or bilateral augmentation implants or injection for bilateral vocal paresis.

Consults
- Otolaryngology
- Speech and swallow therapy

Complications of treatment
- Airway edema and hematoma are major complications of airway surgery
- Implant migration
- Poor voice

Prognosis
- Reduction of aspiration and improved quality of voice can be attained with appropriate therapy or surgical intervention.

Helpful Hints
- While treatment is indicated immediately upon diagnosis, it is wise to delay irreversible surgery for about 6 months in cases in which recovery of the recurrent laryngeal nerve is a possibility.

Suggested Readings
Merati AL, Heman-Ackah YD, Abaza M, Altman KW, Sulica L, Belamowicz S. Common movement disorders affecting the larynx: a report from the neurolaryngology committee of the AAO-HNS. *Otolaryngol Head Neck Surg.* 2005;i33(5):654–655.
Richardson BE, Bastian RW. Clinical evaluation of vocal fold paralysis. *Otolaryngol Clin North Am.* 2004;37(1):45–58.
Rubin AD, Sataloff RT. Vocal fold paresis and paralysis. *Otolaryngol Clin North Am.* 2007;40(5):1109–1131.

Section I: Conditions

Autonomic Nervous System Issues: Autonomic Dysreflexia

Jung-Woo Ma MD ■ Thomas N. Bryce MD

Description
Autonomic dysreflexia (AD) is a condition of imbalanced reflex sympathetic discharge in response to noxious stimuli after SCI.

Etiology/Types
- Reactive to noxious stimuli below the level of injury
- Reactive to central nervous system abnormality such as syringomyelia
- Idiopathic

Epidemiology
- All individuals with complete injuries above T6 can have symptoms of AD with a sufficient stimulus
- Occurs in persons with either complete or incomplete SCI
- Symptoms are less common and severe in persons with incomplete SCI
- Rarely occurs in persons with lesions below T6
- Does not occur until spinal shock has resolved

Pathogenesis
- A noxious stimulus activates nociceptors below the level of the lesion setting off a barrage of afferent impulses.
- Sympathetic neurons are activated in the spinal cord below the level of the lesion producing a generalized sympathetic response.
- The generalized sympathetic response generates increased peripheral resistance, circulating blood volume, and an elevation in blood pressure.
- Inhibitory signals generated by brain stem vasomotor centers are unable to descend (when the injury level is at T6 or above) to the splanchnic vascular beds, which could accommodate the increased blood volume.
- Parasympathetic output prevails above the injury level leading to nasal congestion, flushing, and sweating above the level of the injury.
- Vasomotor brain stem reflexes attempt to lower blood pressure by increasing vagal parasympathetic stimulation to the heart, causing bradycardia.

Risk Factors
- Bladder distension (75% to 85%)
- Fecal impaction (13% to 19%)
- Pressure ulcers
- Urinary tract infection (UTI)
- Ingrown toenails
- Menstruation
- Labor and delivery
- Cholecystitis
- Gastric ulcers or gastritis
- Hemorrhoids
- Sexual activity
- Constrictive clothing
- Fractures or other trauma
- Detrusor sphincter dyssynergia
- Syringomyelia

Clinical Features
- Pounding headache
- Hypertension
- Profuse sweating and flushing above the level of injury
- Blurry vision

Natural History
- A noxious enough stimulus can produce AD in almost anyone with a high thoracic or cervical SCI.
- Untreated severe hypertension accompanying AD may lead to retinal hemorrhage, cerebral hemorrhage, seizures, and death.

Diagnosis

Differential diagnosis
- Essential hypertension
- Pheochromocytoma
- Migraine and cluster headaches
- Toxemia of pregnancy

History
- Acute onset of severe headache, blurry vision, nasal congestion, and sweating

Exam
- Sudden rise in blood pressure, generally >20 mm Hg

- Profuse sweating, piloerection, and flushing above the level of lesion
- Bradycardia

Testing
- Blood pressure and pulse monitoring
- Abdominal flat plate to look for impaction
- Urinalysis and urine culture if urinary tract infection is suspected
- MRI of cervical spine if no cause can be found

Pitfalls
- Failure to recognize mild symptoms, especially headache, as AD
- Failure to recognize that baseline blood pressure can be quite low in persons with tetraplegia and resultant increase to a seemingly modest absolute blood pressure may be quite a significant increase

Red Flags
- Chest pain
- New neurologic dysfunction

Treatment

Medical
- Sit patient upright
- Loosen clothing
- Relieve obstruction to drainage of an indwelling urinary catheter
- If no indwelling catheter present then catheterize patient
- If the systolic blood pressure is still ≥150 mm Hg, administer rapidly acting and easily reversible antihypertensives, such as topical nitroglycerin ointment
- If the systolic blood pressure is <150 mm Hg, then the rectum should be manually disimpacted

- Search for other precipitants if symptoms persist
- Prophylactic treatment for patients with recurrent episodes of AD can include alpha blockade or ganglion blockade
- Use of a local anesthetic gel can help prevent AD triggered by digital stimulation or urethral catheterization

Consults
- Physical medicine and rehabilitation
- Neurourology
- Gastroenterology

Complications of treatment
- Hypotension from antihypertensives

Prognosis
- The condition can nearly always be managed successfully if underlying cause can be identified and eliminated.
- Mortality is rare.

Helpful Hints
- Patients should be educated about the clinical findings and treatment for this condition.

Suggested Readings

Blackmer J. Rehabilitation medicine. 1. Autonomic dysreflexia. *CMAJ.* 2003;169(9):931–935.

Bryce TN, Ragnarsson KT. Spinal cord injury. In: Braddom RL, ed. *Physical Medicine & Rehabilitation.* 3rd ed. Boston: Saunders Elsevier; 2007:1325–1326.

Bycroft J, Shergill IS, Choong EAL, Arya N, Shah PJR. Autonomic dysreflexia: a medical emergency. *Postgrad Med J.* 2005;81:232–235.

McLachlan EM. Diversity of sympathetic vasoconstrictor pathways and their plasticity after spinal cord injury. *Clin Auton Res.* 2007;17:6–12.

Autonomic Nervous System Issues: Bradycardia

Matthew M. Shatzer DO

Description

Bradycardia is defined as a drop in heart rate below 60 beats per minute (bpm), although it typically is not symptomatic until it falls below 40 to 50 bpm. Bradycardia is one of the clinical manifestations of neurogenic shock, which occurs shortly after SCI. It occurs in almost all persons with complete tetraplegia.

Etiology/Types

■ Unopposed parasympathetic input to the heart

Epidemiology

■ Potentially occurs in all persons with tetraplegia
■ Rare during chronic phase of SCI except during episodes of intense vagal stimulation, as observed in response to an episode of autonomic dysreflexia

Pathogenesis

■ Sympathetic input to the heart, which originates from the T1 to T4 spinal levels, is interrupted when the SCI occurs to the cervical or upper thoracic spine.
■ Parasympathetic control of the heart, which originates in the medulla, is not affected by the injury to the spinal cord as it is carried by the vagus nerve.
■ An imbalance occurs in which there is unopposed parasympathetic input to the heart, resulting in bradycardia.
■ Other mechanisms that can induce bradycardia include tracheobronchial suctioning, defecation, and belching, which can cause sinus pauses and unopposed parasympathetic activity.

Risk Factors

■ Cervical or high thoracic SCI
■ Complete cervical or high thoracic SCI

Clinical Features

■ Dizziness
■ Syncope
■ Fatigue

Natural History

■ Bradycardia is most pronounced during the first 2 weeks following injury.

■ If untreated, it can progress to cardiac arrest or severe atrioventricular block.
■ Heart rate usually returns to baseline by 6 weeks.

Diagnosis

Differential diagnosis

■ Myocardial infarct
■ Myocarditis
■ Medication effect
■ Heart block
■ Cardiomyopathy
■ Electrolyte abnormality
■ An efficient heart with resting bradycardia

History

■ Typically noted by medical staff upon initial evaluation
■ Person may experience dizziness, lightheadedness, weakness, and fatigue
■ Loss of consciousness

Exam

■ Heart rate <60 bpm
■ Hypotension

Testing

■ Electrocardiogram (EKG)
■ Continuous cardiac monitoring
■ Serum chemistry

Pitfalls

■ Hypoxia or manipulation of the larynx or trachea can cause profound bradycardia or even cardiac arrest in persons with high tetraplegia.

Red Flags

■ Loss of consciousness
■ Profound hypotension

Treatment

Medical

■ Observation without intervention is indicated if there is no hemodynamic compromise

- Atropine 0.5 to 1 mg intravenously (may be given 1 to 5 minutes before suctioning or airway manipulation)
- Vasopressors, ideally with both alpha- and beta-adrenergic actions (ie, dopamine, norepinephrine, epinephrine)
- Transvenous temporary pacing

Surgical
- Permanent pacemaker

Consults
- Cardiology, if bradycardia is severe or persistent.

Complications of treatment
- Hypertension
- Tachycardia
- Surgical site infections associated with placement of transvenous or permanent pacemakers

Prognosis
- Bradycardia should resolve spontaneously within 6 weeks after injury.
- Permanent pacing is rarely required.

Helpful Hints
- Presence of bradycardia differentiates neurogenic shock from hypovolemic shock, which would present with tachycardia.
- Cardiovascular interventions, such as vasopressors, atropine, aminophylline, or pacemakers, are more commonly required in individuals with high cervical injury.

Suggested Readings

Campagnolo DI, Merli GJ. Autonomic and cardiovascular complications of spinal cord injury. In: Kirshblum S, Campagnolo DI, DeLisa JA, eds. *Spinal Cord Medicine*. Philadelphia: Lippincott Williams & Wilkins; 2002:123–134.

Consortium for spinal cord medicine et al. Early acute management in adults with spinal cord injury: a clinical practice guideline for heath-care professionals. *J Spinal Cord Med*. 2008;31(4):403–479.

Lehmann KG, Lane JG, Piepmeier JM, et al. Cardiovascular abnormalities accompanying acute spinal cord injury in humans: incidence, time course and severity. *J Am Coll Cardiol*. 1987;10(1):46–52.

Section I: Conditions

Autonomic Nervous System Issues: Orthostatic Hypotension

Matthew M. Shatzer DO

Description
Orthostatic hypotension is a decrease in systolic blood pressure of >20 mm Hg and/or a decrease in diastolic blood pressure of >10 mm Hg, when changing from the supine to an upright position.

Etiology/Types
- Pooling of blood in the lower extremities and viscera, in combination with an inadequate response by the cardiovascular system, results in orthostasis

Epidemiology
- Exact incidence in SCI is not known but it is more common in higher levels of injury, particularly complete injuries.

Pathogenesis
- Orthostatic hypotension is a condition that occurs due to a disruption of efferent sympathetic activity.
- In an able-bodied individual, the pooling of blood that occurs with positional changes is counteracted by sympathetic outflow and resultant vasoconstriction and tachycardia.
- Since sympathetic outflow is interrupted in the spinal cord-injured individual, there is a loss of vascular resistance with resultant accumulation of blood within the venous system and reduced return to the heart.
- In an able-bodied individual, the carotid baroceptor responds to a loss of vascular resistance. However, this mechanism is interrupted in the high spinal cord-injured individual, which further exacerbates the hypotension.

Risk Factors
- Injury level above T6
- Complete SCI

Clinical Features
- Dizziness, feeling faint
- Syncope
- Nausea
- Fatigue
- Pallor
- Perioral and facial numbness
- Poor tolerance of upright position and restorative therapies

Natural History
Tends to improve gradually over time in early rehabilitation period due to the following factors:
- Restoration of fluid balance
- Improved autoregulation of cerebral circulation
- Improved sensitivity of baroreceptor wall
- Adaptation of plasma renin-angiotensin system
- Development of spasticity that improves venous return

Diagnosis

Differential diagnosis
- Volume depletion
- Medication effect
- Post-traumatic cystic myelopathy
- Myocardial infarction, cardiomyopathy
- Adrenal insufficiency

History
- Dizziness or loss of consciousness when going from supine to sit or sit to stand
- Dizziness associated with meals
- Poor tolerance of therapy with easy fatigability

Exam
- Greater than 20 mm Hg drop in systolic blood pressure and/or a greater than 10 mm Hg decrease in diastolic blood pressure when changing from supine to upright position
- Absence of compensatory tachycardia

Testing
- Blood count and chemistry to evaluate for volume depletion
- EKG to rule out myocardial infarction
- Tilt table testing

Pitfalls
- Must exclude other reversible causes of hypotension such as anemia, vascular depletion, adrenal insufficiency, or medications.

- Volume enhancing medications must be used with caution in individuals with cardiac insufficiency.
- Patients susceptible to autonomic dysreflexia must be monitored closely if being treated with sympathomimetics as these may potentiate a markedly elevated blood pressure during a dysreflexic episode.

Red Flags
- Syncope
- Bradycardia

Treatment

Medical
- Elastic abdominal binder
- Lower limb compression stockings
- Decrease seat-back angle in a recliner wheelchair from near supine gradually to full upright as tolerated
- Gradually increase head of bed before getting out of bed
- Salt tablets: 1 to 2 g two to three times daily, before meals
- Fludrocortisone: 0.1 to 0.3 mg one to two times per day
- Midodrine: 2.5 to 5 mg one to three times per day
- Ephedrine: 20 to 30 mg one to four times daily

Exercises
- Tilt table

Modalities
- Electrical stimulation of leg muscles

Consults
- Cardiology, if persistent

Complications of treatment
- Hypertension, tachycardia from sympathomimetics
- Fluid retention, edema, and hypokalemia from mineralcorticoids
- Pressure ulcers from compression garments

Prognosis
- Generally resolves over time without long-term need for medical treatments.

Helpful Hints
- May attempt adrenocorticotropic hormone stimulation test to evaluate for adrenal insufficiency
- Monitor for rebound hypertension with pharmacologic treatment

Suggested Readings

Campagnolo DI, Merli GJ. Autonomic and cardiovascular complications of spinal cord injury. In: Kirshblum S, Campagnolo DI, DeLisa JA, eds. *Spinal Cord Medicine*. Philadelphia: Lippincott Williams & Wilkins; 2002:123–134.

Consortium for Spinal Cord Medicine et al. Early acute management in adults with spinal cord injury: a clinical practice guideline for health care professionals. *J Spinal Cord Med.* 2008;31(4):403–479.

Teasell RW, Arnold JMO, Krassioukov A, Delaney GA. Cardiovascular consequences of loss of supraspinal control of the sympathetic nervous system after spinal cord injury. *Arch Phys Med Rehabil.* 2000;81(4):506–516.

Autonomic Nervous System Issues: Spinal Shock

Kristjan T. Ragnarsson MD ■ Thomas N. Bryce MD

Description

Spinal or neurogenic shock refers to the temporary absence or reduction of spinal reflex activity below the neurological level beginning immediately after a SCI. Spinal shock resolves through a series of four phases that correspond to the return of reflex activity.

Etiology/Types

- Spinal shock with significant hypotension and bradycardia
- Spinal shock without significant hypotension and bradycardia

Epidemiology

- Develops in all persons with acute SCI but tends to occur with significant hypotension and bradycardia only in those with neurologically complete lesions above T6

Pathogenesis

Phase 1: areflexia/hyporeflexia

- Spinal neuron hyperpolarization
- Loss of normal background descending excitatory input (serotonergic and noradrenergic neurons especially) to spinal neurons
- Loss of tonic descending facilitation of gamma-motor neurons regulating muscle spindles
- Increased spinal inhibition
- Sympathetic denervation
- Peripheral vasodilatation and reduced peripheral vascular resistance can result in hypotension with diminished venous blood return to the heart and reduced cardiac output
- Insufficient sympathetic activity and unopposed parasympathetic stimulation can cause bradycardia

Phase 2: initial reflex return

- Denervation supersensitivity to neurotransmitters
- Receptor up-regulation in motor neurons

Phase 3: initial hyper-reflexia

- Axon supported synapse growth

Phase 4: final hyper-reflexia

- Soma-supported synapse growth

Risk Factors

- Neurologic level above T6
- Complete injury [American Spinal Injury Association (ASIA) Impairment Scale level A]

Clinical Features

Phase 1

- Occurs 0 to 1 day after injury
- Absence of deep tendon reflexes (DTRs)
- Recovery of the cutaneous polysynaptic reflexes: delayed plantar reflex, cremasteric reflex, bulbocavernosis reflex, and anocutaneous reflex
- Hypotension
- Bradycardia can be aggravated by tracheal suctioning and bowel activity
- Hypothermia
- Cardiac arrest is rare

Phase 2

- Occurs 1 to 3 days after injury
- Recovery of DTRs can occur although they are typically absent
- Recovery of Babinski sign can occur although it is typically absent
- Stronger cutaneous polysynaptic reflexes

Phase 3

- Occurs 4 to 30 days after injury
- Most DTRs reappear as well as Babinski sign
- Autonomic function improves with improvement of bradycardia and hypotension
- Autonomic dysreflexia can emerge

Phase 4

- Occurs 1 to 12 months after injury
- Cutaneous reflexes and DTRs become hyperactive
- Detrusor reflexes often begin by 4 to 6 weeks

Natural History

- Progress through the four phases can be slower in those who are elderly, frail, or have an infection or other secondary illness
- Vasovagal hypotension and bradyarrythmias typically resolve by 3 to 6 weeks

Diagnosis

Differential diagnosis
- Hypovolemic shock (increased systemic vascular resistance)
- Other causes of hemodynamic instability

Exam
- Areflexia or hyporeflexia
- Hypotension
- Variable heart rate

Testing
- For spinal shock with significant hypotension and bradycardia, monitor mean arterial blood pressure, pulmonary capillary wedge pressure, and cardiac output by pulmonary artery catheterization

Pitfalls
- Hypovolemic shock and spinal shock can be confused leading to serious mismanagement; hypovolemic shock requires fluid replacement while spinal shock with decreased systemic vascular resistance requires vasopressor administration.

Red Flags
- Sustained hypotension with diminished urinary output
- Severe bradycardia (<30 bpm)

Treatment

Medical
- Administer vasopressors, for example, dopamine, phenylnephrine, or phentolamine for significant hypotension (after intravascular volume is restored)
- For significant bradycardia, administer anticholinergic agents (eg, atropine)
- Place temporary transvenous or transcutaneous cardiac pacemaker

Surgical
- Place a permanent cardiac pacemaker if significant bradycardia lasts >6 weeks

Consults
- Cardiology

Complications of treatment
- Unnecessary placement of permanent pacemaker

Prognosis
- Hypotension may reduce blood flow to the spinal cord and affect the neurologic outcome.
- Significant hypotension and bradycardia usually resolve spontaneously.

Helpful Hints
- Permanent cardiac pacemaker is rarely necessary.
- If spinal shock is defined as the absence of all reflex activity, then it probably lasts less than an hour in most cases.
- If spinal shock is defined as the absence of all DTRs, then it probably lasts several weeks.

Suggested Readings
Arkinson PP, Arkinson JL. Spinal shock. *Mayo Clin Proc.* 1996;71:384–389.

Consortium for Spinal Cord Medicine. Early acute management in adults with spinal cord injury: a clinical practice guideline for health-care professionals. *J Spinal Cord Med.* 2008;31(4):403–479.

Ditunno JF, Little JW, Tessler A, Burns AS. Spinal shock revisited: a four-phase model. *Spinal Cord.* 2004;42(7):383–395.

Piepmeier JM, Lehmann KB, Lane JG. Cardiovascular instability following acute cervical spinal cord trauma. *Cent Nerv Syst Trauma.* 1985;2:153–160.

Section I: Conditions

Autonomic Nervous System Issues: Thermal Dysregulation and Fever

Kristjan T. Ragnarsson MD

Description

Impaired regulation of core body temperature is especially prevalent in persons with neurologically complete SCI above T6 neurologic level.

Etiology/Types

- Fever after acute SCI (neurogenic or "quad" fever)
- Chronic thermal deregulation

Epidemiology

- Greatest prevalence in persons with neurologically complete lesions above T6

Pathogenesis

- Loss of hypothalamic supraspinal control over peripheral temperature modifying mechanisms
- Normally body temperature is primarily controlled by the hypothalamus and secondarily by personal behavior to increase or decrease heat loss
- As core body temperature rises or falls, thermal regulation normally occurs by activation or inhibition of the sympathetic nervous system, that is, vasoconstriction and shivering for heat preservation and sweating to increase heat loss.
- High level, complete SCI results in loss of supraspinal control over the sympathetic nervous system and thus over vasomotor activity, sweating, shivering, and so on.
- Persons with SCI tend to be poikilothermic, that is, have relatively high temperature in warm environments and low temperature in cold environments.

Risk Factors

- High level neurologically complete SCI

Clinical Features

- Persistent fever after an acute SCI without identifiable source
- Subnormal body temperature in cold environment (body temperature <37°C)
- Elevated body temperature in warm environment and during increased metabolic activity, eg, physical exercise, acute trauma, and illnesses.

- Most of the time, persons with SCI maintain normal or near-normal body temperature by their conscious or unconscious behavior.
- Degree of thermal dysregulation may vary depending on neurologic level and completeness of cord lesion

Natural History

- People with high-level neurologically complete SCI do not regain central thermoregulatory control, although the persistent fever after acute SCI usually resolves spontaneously.
- People with low-level SCI (below T6) are rarely clinically affected.
- People with neurologically incomplete SCI may regain central thermoregulatory control to a varying degree.

Diagnosis

Differential diagnosis

- Fever due to infection, including but not limited to sinusitis, cellulitis, osteomyelitis, bronchitis, pneumonia, cholecystitis, pancreatitis, pyelonephritis, *Clostridium difficile* colitis, cystitis, epididymitis, and prostatitis
- Thermal deregulation due to thyroid dysfunction
- Fever due to inflammatory conditions including but not limited to pulmonary embolus, bowel infarction, stool impaction, heterotopic ossification, deep venous thrombosis, cancer, and occult long bone fractures.

History

- Fever after an acute SCI without infectious, inflammatory, or other identifiable source
- Fluctuating body temperature related to environmental temperature, physical activity, and so on

Exam

- Perform complete physical exam survey looking for potential causes of fever or inflammation

Testing

- Complete blood count, erythrocyte sedimentation rate, C-reactive protein, thyroid function tests, blood cultures, urinalysis, and culture

- CT with contrast of the chest, abdomen, and pelvis, to look for an infectious source of fever when the history and physical exam are unremarkable in the acute setting
- A labeled white blood cell scan can be useful for identifying an occult infection
- A duplex ultrasound of the legs to evaluate for deep venous thrombosis
- CT or MRI with contrast of the spine to evaluate for osteomyelitis or spinal abscess

Pitfalls

- Hastily attributing elevated body temperature after acute SCI to temperature dysregulation ("quad fever")

Red Flags

- Hypotension
- Elevated white blood cell count

Treatment

Medical

- Rule out infectious cause
- Proper heating and cooling of environment
- Wear clothes appropriate for the weather and for the environment.
- Avoid strenuous exercise in hot environment.
- Apply cool, moist compresses with rising body temperatures.

Consults

- Infectious disease

Complications of treatment

- Masking of underlying cause

Prognosis

- Fever of no identifiable cause after acute SCI generally resolves spontaneously.
- Thermal deregulation is permanent after high complete SCI.
- Thermal deregulation may improve after incomplete SCI.

Helpful Hints

- Neurogenic cause of fever is a diagnosis of exclusion.
- Atelectasis in patients with high level SCI often is an unrecognized cause of fever misattributed to neurogenic or quad fever.

Suggested Readings

Cesario TC, Darouiche RO. Thermal regulation in the SCI patient. In: Lin VW, ed. *Spinal Cord Medicine Principles and Practice*. New York: Demos; 2003:209–211.

Mallory BS. Autonomic function in the isolated spinal cord. In: Gonzales EG, et al., eds. *Downey and Darlings Physiological Basis of Rehabilitation Medicine*. Boston: Butterworth Heinemann; 2001:683–710.

Section I: Conditions

Bladder Dysfunction: Lower Motor Neuron

Silvia G. Geraci DO ■ Adam B. Stein MD

Description
Injury to the spinal cord at or below the sacral micturition center (S2–S4), including the conus medullaris and/or cauda equina, results in an areflexic or hyporeflexic bladder.

Etiology/Types
- Trauma to conus/cauda
- Lumbar central disc herniation
- Primary or metastatic tumors
- Myelodysplasia
- Arteriovenous malformation
- Arachnoiditis

Epidemiology
- In one series, traumatic spinal injury was the cause of lower motor neuron (LMN) bladder dysfunction in over 50% of individuals.

Pathogenesis
- The sacral reflex arc is disrupted and blocks parasympathetic transmission to the detrusor muscle, resulting in weak or absent bladder contractions.
- Pelvic nerve innervation to the bladder typically arises one segment rostral to the pudendal innervation to the sphincter; therefore, the external urethral sphincter is usually not affected to the same extent as the bladder.
- SCI at this level leads to detrusor areflexia and a relatively competent sphincter resulting in bladder overdistention.
- Detrusor areflexia may be accompanied by reduced bladder compliance resulting in a gradual increase in intravesical pressure with bladder filling.

Risk Factors
- SCI or disease involving the conus medullaris or cauda equina

Clinical Features
- Urinary retention
- Overflow incontinence
- Abdominal distention
- Constipation

Natural History
- Uncompensated LMN bladder produces urinary retention that can lead to overflow or stress incontinence
- Recurrent UTIs
- Bladder or kidney stones
- Vesicoureteral reflux, hydronephrosis, and renal disease less likely than in upper motor neuron (UMN) bladder

Diagnosis
Differential diagnosis
- Spinal shock
- Multiple sclerosis
- Obstructive uropathy
- Syringomyelia
- Autonomic neuropathies (eg, Shy-Drager syndrome)
- Tabes dorsalis
- Pernicious anemia

History
- Urinary retention
- Abdominal straining to initiate voiding
- Weak stream with voiding
- Stress incontinence
- Constipation

Exam
- Lower abdominal distention with palpable firm bladder
- Abdominal tenderness
- Absent sacral reflexes
- Associated LMN signs (muscle atrophy, depressed or absent deep tendon reflexes)

Testing
- High postvoid residual urine
- Urodynamic study

Pitfalls
- Need to differentiate from UMN bladder

Red Flags
- Hematuria
- Change in typical bladder pattern

Treatment

Medical

- Intermittent catheterization is the preferred method of management
- Crede and Valsalva maneuvers allow for a degree of bladder emptying that may obviate need for catheterization
- Condom catheter may be useful for a man with associated uncontrollable stress incontinence
- Fluid restriction
- Bethanechol hydrochloride may be tried, but supporting literature is limited

Exercises

- Kegel exercises may help minimize associated stress incontinence.

Modalities

- Persons with LMN bladders are not candidates for electrical stimulation of the detrusor to initiate voiding.

Surgical

- Suprapubic catheter if sphincter mechanism is competent and intermittent catheterization is not an achievable option.
- Artificial sphincter to resolve severe stress incontinence

Consults

- Neurourology

Complications of treatment

- Urethral trauma, including urethral erosions, false passages, and fistulas from catheterization
- Hernias, hemorrhoids, or rectal prolapse from Credé and Valsalva maneuvers
- Side effects of bethanechol include diarrhea, bradycardia, excess salivation, and tearing

Prognosis

- Incomplete lesions have a greater likelihood of regaining bladder continence.
- With the appropriate treatment and surveillance, patients can be expected to find a method of bladder management that will minimize medical complications.

Helpful Hints

- There is a higher incidence of bladder cancer with indwelling catheters.
- Hand dexterity, caregiver assistance, and mobility must be considered when choosing an appropriate bladder regimen.

Suggested Readings

Consortium for Spinal Cord Medicine et al. Bladder management for adults with spinal cord injury. *J Spinal Cord Med.* 2006;29(5):527–573.

Gillenwater JY, Grayhack JT, Howards SS, et al., eds. *Adult and Pediatric Urology.* 4th ed. Philadelphia: Lippincott, Williams & Wilkins; 2002.

Pavlakis AJ, Siroky, MB, Goldstein I, et al. Neurourologic findings in conus medullaris and cauda equine injury. *Arch Neurol.* 1983;40:570–573.

Section I: Conditions

Bladder Dysfunction: Upper Motor Neuron

Silvia G. Geraci DO ■ Adam B. Stein MD

Description
Injury to the spinal cord above the sacral micturition center results in a hyper-reflexic neurogenic bladder.

Etiology/Types
■ UMN bladder with coordinated sphincter
■ UMN bladder with detrusor sphincter dyssynergia (DSD)

Epidemiology
■ 96% of persons with UMN bladder in SCI develop DSD.

Pathogenesis
■ The sacral micturition reflex arc remains intact, enabling bladder contraction with filling.
■ The inhibitory effect of the cerebral cortex on the sacral micturition center is blocked by the cord lesion leading to involuntary bladder contractions.
■ DSD is the failure of the sphincter to relax during bladder contraction due to interruption of the coordinating effect of the pontine micturition center.
■ Sympathetic efferents (T11-L2) are typically affected, further inhibiting bladder storage and favoring an overactive bladder pattern.

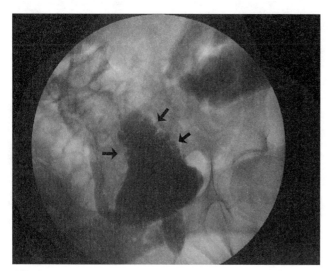

"Christmas tree" bladder. The hypertrophied detrusor muscle outlined by the arrows has taken on the appearance of a Christmas tree.

Risk Factors
■ SCI or disease above the sacral micturition center

Clinical Features
■ Urinary incontinence
■ Uninhibited bladder contractions causing abdominal pain or discomfort
■ "Stop/start voiding" with incomplete emptying (in DSD)

Natural History
■ DSD occurs in virtually everyone with an UMN bladder
■ Vesicoureteral reflux, hydronephrosis, and renal disease
■ Recurrent UTIs
■ Bladder or kidney stones
■ Autonomic dysreflexia in T6 or higher SCI

Diagnosis

Differential diagnosis
■ Cord lesions
  – Multiple sclerosis
  – Neuromyelitis optica
  – Spinal tumors
  – Transverse myelitis
  – Epidural abscess
  – Spondylotic myelopathy
  – Vascular malformations
■ Suprapontine lesions
  – Parkinsons disease
  – Multiple sclerosis
  – Normal pressure hydrocephalus
  – Intracranial neoplasms
  – Stroke/brain injury

History
■ Urge incontinence unrelated to body position

Exam
■ UMN signs including hyper-reflexia, spasticity
■ Intact bulbocavernosus reflex and anocutaneous reflex (anal wink)

Testing
■ Postvoid residual urine measurement
■ Urodynamic study

Pitfalls
- Need to differentiate between UMN and LMN bladder, as both can present with incontinence

Red Flags
- Rising creatinine
- Autonomic dysreflexia during voiding
- Pyelonephritis

Treatment

Medical
- Anticholinergics (eg, oxybutynin, tolteradine)
- Alpha-blockers (eg, tamsulosin, doxazosin)
- Intermittent catheterization (IC)
- Condom catheter for males only with "balanced bladder" characterized by low voiding pressure and complete bladder emptying
- Indwelling catheters

Exercises
- Avoid Credé and Valsalva maneuvers

Modalities
- Anterior sacral root stimulation, with posterior rhizotomies provides actual bladder control via neurostimulation

Injection
- Botulinum toxin into sphincter or bladder wall for persons with DSD

Surgical
- Suprapubic cystostomy
- Transurethral sphincterotomy, males only
- Endourethral stents, males only
- Posterior sacral rhizotomy + IC
- Augmentation cystoplasty + IC

Consults
- Physical medicine and rehabilitation
- Neurourology

Complications of treatment
- Skin breakdown, pressure ulcers, urethral trauma with hematuria from catheters
- Sacral rhizotomy is irreversible and will lead to loss of reflex erection, reflex ejaculation, and sacral sensation

Prognosis
- With treatment and surveillance, people can find an acceptable bladder regimen that minimizes medical complications and provides a socially acceptable method of bladder drainage.
- Persons with motor incomplete SCI are more likely to regain urinary control than those with complete injuries.

Helpful Hints
- Caregiver assistance and individual preferences should be strongly considered when prescribing a method of bladder management.
- Combination therapy is common including IC with anticholinergics and condom catheter with alpha blockers.
- There is a higher incidence of bladder cancer with indwelling catheters than without.

Suggested Readings
Consortium for spinal cord medicine et al. Clinical practice guidelines: Bladder management for adults with spinal cord injury. *J Spinal Cord Med.* 2006;29(5):527–573.

Federle M, Jeffrey RB, Anne VS, et al. *Diagnostic Imaging Abdomen.* Amirsys; 2004.

Gillenwater JY, Grayhack JT, Howards SS, et al., eds. *Adult and Pediatric Urology.* 4th ed. Philadelphia: Lippincott Williams & Wilkins; 2002.

Lin VW, Cardenas DD, et al., eds. *Spinal Cord Medicine:Principles and Practice.* New York: Demos; 2003.

Bladder Dysfunction: Urinary Tract Infections

Silvia G. Geraci DO ■ Adam B. Stein MD

Description
UTI is the presence of significant bacteriuria associated with pyuria and related signs or symptoms.

Etiology/Types
- Cystitis
- Pyelonephritis

Epidemiology
- UTI is common among persons with SCI.
- Within 6 weeks of SCI, 46% of persons using catheters develop UTI.
- Twenty percent annual incidence of UTI in SCI.
- Persons with indwelling catheters have higher rates of UTI than those using intermittent catheterization or condom catheters.
- After 4 days of indwelling catheter use, 100% of individuals will develop bacteriuria.
- 2% to 4% of persons with catheter-associated bacteriuria will develop bacteremia.

Pathogenesis
- Most common organisms are Gram-negative bacilli and enterococci.
- Catheterization can introduce bacteria directly into the urinary tract.
- Urinary stasis provides a medium in which bacteria thrive.

Risk Factors
- Catheter use leading to chronic bacterial colonization
- Incomplete bladder emptying
- Catheter occlusion
- Detrusor-sphincter dyssynergia (DSD)
- Vesicoureteral reflux
- Urinary tract stones
- Needing assistance for bladder care
- Fecal incontinence

Clinical Features
- Fever
- Cloudy, bloody, or foul-smelling urine

- Incontinence when previously continent on intermittent catheterization
- Increased spasticity
- Autonomic dysreflexia, in susceptible persons

Natural History
- Most UTIs can be avoided by appropriate bladder management and monitoring for signs and symptoms.
- Appropriate antibiotic therapy successfully treats most UTIs.
- Untreated UTIs can progress to pyelonephritis, bacteremia, and perinephric abcess.

Diagnosis

Differential diagnosis
- Asymptomatic bacteriuria
- Pyelonephritis
- Cystitis
- Detrusor hyperreflexia

History
- Frequency, urgency, dysuria
- Onset of urinary incontinence when previously continent
- Bladder spasms
- Autonomic dysreflexia

Exam
- Fever
- Increased spasticity
- Suprapubic or flank discomfort
- Cloudy, bloody, or malodorous urine

Testing
- Urinalysis: significant bacteriuria ($\geq 10^4$ CFU/mL for clean-void specimens from males using condom catheters; or $\geq 10^2$ CFU/mL for catheter specimens) or pyuria (>10^4 WBC/mL of uncentrifuged urine or >10 WBC/hpf of spun urine)
- Positive urine culture

Pitfalls
- Frequency, urgency, dysuria, and flank tenderness are often absent in persons with SCI.

- Treating asymptomatic bacteriuria can lead to development of antibiotic-resistant organisms.
- Carefully evaluate persons with SCI and fever to exclude other potential causes not appreciated in light of sensory deficit.

Red Flags
- Beware of signs and symptoms of urosepsis, which may include high fever, hypotension, high white blood cell count, tachycardia, tachypnea, and/or change in mental status. This can be life-threatening if not treated rapidly.

Treatment

Medical
- Choose antibiotic therapy based upon urine culture
- Consider anticholinergics for bladder spasms
- Catheters should be changed when UTI occurs
- Frequency of intermittent catheterization (IC) may need to be adjusted
- May need to switch from clean technique to sterile IC if recurrent symptomatic UTI

Surgical
- If UTI related to urolithiasis, intervention is warranted for stone eradication.

Consults
- Urology, if recurrent UTI related to DSD, stones, or reflux
- Infectious disease for resistant bacteria requiring broader, more costly antibiotics or for empiric treatment

Complications of treatment
- *Clostridium difficile* colitis
- Allergic reactions and side effects related to antibiotics

Prognosis
- With appropriate bladder management, urologic surveillance, and judicious use of antibiotics, frequency of UTIs should be minimized, and when occurring, should be easy to treat.
- There is a 10% mortality from urinary sepsis.

Helpful Hints
- Specimens can be obtained for culture via sterile procedure to avoid contamination.
- Urine cultures revealing multiple organisms commonly represent contamination and should be repeated.
- Hematuria does not always indicate UTI.
- Use of chronic prophylactic antimicrobials is discouraged to avoid resistance, exceptions may include during pregnancy or perioperative periods.
- Persons with persistent or recurrent UTIs should be evaluated for anatomical anomalies or functional alterations.

Suggested Readings
Jamil E. Towards a catheter free status in neurogenic bladder dysfunction: a review of bladder management options in spinal cord injury (SCI). *Spinal Cord.* 2001;39:355–361.

Leoni MEG, DeRuz AE. Management of urinary tract infection in patients with spinal cord injury. *Clin Microbiol Infect.* 2003;9(8):780–785.

Lin VW, Cardenas DD, Cutter NC, et al., eds. *Spinal Cord Medicine: Principles and Practice.* New York: Demos; 2003.

Section I: Conditions

Bladder Dysfunction: Urolithiasis

Justin T. Hata MD

Description
Stones or calculi that form within the urinary system (kidneys, ureters, or bladder) are a common complication of neurogenic bladder dysfunction in SCI.

Etiology/Types
- Struvite stones: magnesium ammonium phosphate
- Calcium stones (phosphate or oxalate)
- Uric acid stones
- Cystine stones

Epidemiology
- 7% of persons with SCI develop urolithiasis within 10 years of injury.
- Calcium-based stones typically form <2 years post-SCI.
- Greatest risk is during the first 3 to 6 months post-SCI.
- Infection related stones typically form >2 years post-SCI.
- 98% of stones in SCI are either struvite or calcium phosphate.
- Most commonly found in white males with SCI.
- Occurs more frequently in hot, arid areas
- Recurrence rate is approximately 50% within 10 years.

Pathogenesis
- The most important determinant is supersaturation.
- Calcium-based stones typically form due to hypercalciuria after injury and urinary stasis.
- Urease-producing bacteria (*Proteus*, *Klebsiella*, *Pseudomonas*) cause alkaline urine that predisposes to development of struvite stones.

Risk Factors
- Neurogenic bladder dysfunction
- Immobilization hypercalciuria
- Recurrent UTIs
- Indwelling catheters
- Vesicoureteral reflux
- Urinary tract stasis
- Alkaline urine
- Level and completeness of SCI (higher level and complete injury predispose to calculi)

Clinical Features
- Hematuria
- UTI symptoms (stones can mimic)
- Anorexia
- Nausea and/or vomiting
- Abdominal or flank pain; renal colic (in incomplete patients)
- Autonomic dysreflexia
- Renal insufficiency

Natural History
- Small (<4 mm), asymptomatic renal calculi expected to pass within 1 to 2 weeks; 50% become symptomatic within 5 years.
- Urology referral recommended for stones >4 mm or for stones that have not passed after 2 to 4 weeks.
- Staghorn renal calculi are associated with renal damage and require rapid treatment.
- Unrecognized stone disease can lead to renal failure.

Diagnosis

Differential diagnosis
- Renal or urinary tract tumors
- UTI
- Other causes of obstructive uropathy
- Other causes of abdominal pain (eg, appendicitis, diverticulitis, neuropathic pain)

History
- Persons with SCI with significant sensory deficits may have subtle and variable presentation; pain suggesting renal colic is often not present.
- Incomplete SCI: abdominal or referred pain may be present along with gross hematuria and/or symptoms of UTI.

Exam
- Minimal or absent exam findings frequently found
- Abdominal tenderness, costovertebral angle tenderness
- Abdominal guarding and rebound

Testing
- Noncontrast helical CT has become the standard for evaluation of acute urolithiasis
- Renal/bladder ultrasound; most useful screening test

- Abdominal plain radiography may show calcifications; uric acid calculi are radiolucent
- Intravenous excretory urography allows imaging of renal parenchyma, collecting system, and ureters
- Stone component identification

Pitfalls
- Clinical presentation can be subtle in SCI; fatigue and anorexia may be the only presenting symptoms

Red Flags
- Sepsis
- Anuria (ureteral stone in single kidney, bilateral urolithiasis, or reflux anuria)
- Acute renal failure

Treatment

Medical
- Urine alkalization (>7.0) for uric acid or cystine calculi
- Small bladder stones can be dissolved by daily hemiacidrin bladder irrigations
- Coexistent pathology (UTI, neurogenic bladder, metabolic abnormalities) must be addressed to prevent stone recurrence

Surgical
- Large bladder stones are treated cystoscopically using laser lithotripsy.
- Renal pelvis stones <1.5 cm or ureteral stones <1 cm are treated with extracorporeal shock wave lithotripsy (ESWL).

- Percutaneous nephrolithotomy (PCNL) is preferred for stones >2 cm; clearance of fragments is poor if individuals are inactive.
- Ureteral stents may relieve ureteral obstruction.

Consults
- Urology.

Complications
- PCNL has an 8.5% to 20% major complication rate (respiratory arrest, perirenal abscess, hydrothorax).
- ESWL and ureteroscopy associated with ureteral stricture.
- Ureteroscopy has been associated with UTI.
- Irritative lower urinary tract symptoms can occur with stenting.

Prognosis
- With expeditious treatment or stone removal, prognosis is excellent.

Helpful Hints
- Persons with SCI with urolithiasis may be completely asymptomatic.

Suggested Readings
Culkin D, Binins MV. Urolithiasis in spinal cord disorders. In: Lin VW, ed. *Spinal Cord Medicine: Principles and Practices.* New York: Demos; 2003.
Portis A, Sundaram C. Diagnosis and initial management of kidney stones. *Am Fam Physician.* 2001;63(7):1329–1338.

Section I: Conditions

Bladder Dysfunction: Vesicoureteral Reflux and Hydronephrosis

Adam B. Stein MD

Description

Vesicoureteral reflux refers to backup of urine from the bladder toward the kidneys. Hydronephrosis is the dilatation of the kidneys' collecting system caused by obstruction to urine flow. Persons with SCI are at risk for reflux and hydronephrosis.

Etiology

- Unrelieved urinary retention
- High pressure voiding resulting from detrusor-sphincter dyssynergia (DSD)
- A poorly compliant bladder
- An obstructing stone in the kidney or ureter
- Chronic bladder wall thickening causing ureteropelvic junction obstruction

Epidemiology

- It is unclear what percentage of persons with SCI with bladder dysfunction develop reflux and hydronephrosis overall.
- 96% of persons with suprasacral spinal cord lesions will develop DSD and are at risk for reflux and hydronephrosis.
- Of individuals with SCI followed by the model systems who underwent renal testing by any method, abnormalities were noted in 6%.

Pathogenesis

- Coordination between detrusor contraction and external sphincter relaxation is directed by the pontine micturition center (PMC).
- An SCI interrupts the spinal pathways between the PMC and the detrusor, disrupting this coordination.
- Reflex detrusor contraction then occurs while the sphincter remains contracted, resulting in high pressure voiding and a functional partial obstruction.
- This sustained high pressure voiding is the primary cause of reflux and hydronephrosis.

Risk Factors

- DSD
- Poor detrusor compliance

- Intravesical pressure >40 cm H_2O on a urodynamic study
- Bladder wall hypertrophy
- Nephrolithiasis
- Recurrent cystitis

Clinical Features

- Persons with SCI who develop reflux and hydronephrosis are most often asymptomatic.
- Can be a cause of unexplained autonomic dysreflexia (AD)
- Significant renal damage caused by hydronephrosis can manifest with signs and symptoms of uremia.

Natural History

- Left untreated, hydronephrosis can progress to renal insufficiency and failure.
- In the 1960s, death rate from renal causes in SCI was reported to be between 37% and 76%.

Diagnosis

Differential diagnosis

- Tumors of the genitourinary system
- Extrinsic compression by tumors, adenopathy, hematoma
- Ureteral anatomic abnormalities (stricture, stenosis, kinks)
- Congenital ureteral valves
- Retrocaval ureter
- Prostate hypertrophy with obstruction
- Trauma

History

- Usually asymptomatic
- Symptoms of AD can be present particularly during voiding
- Recurrent symptomatic UTI

Exam

- No characteristic physical exam findings
- Hematuria can occur with an obstructing stone
- Signs of AD are possible including paroxysmal hypertension, flushing, sweating

Testing
- Renal ultrasound is preferred screening test, recommended at least annually for patients with SCI.
- Supplemental testing can include
  - Urodynamics
  - Renal scan
  - Cystogram
  - Intravenous pyelogram
  - CT scan

Pitfalls
- Frequency of asymptomatic reflux and hydronephrosis makes regular surveillance critical.

Red Flags
- Rising serum creatinine
- Intravesical pressures regularly >40 cm H_2O

Treatment
- Treatment of reflux and hydronephrosis is based on removing or minimizing the inciting stimulus.

Medical
- Anticholinergic agents reduce intravesical pressure
- Alpha blockers reduce functional bladder neck obstruction
- Intermittent catheterization (with anticholinergics)
- Indwelling catheter (urethral or suprapubic)

Injections
- Injection of botulinum toxin into the detrusor or sphincter

Surgery
- Endourethral stents
- Transurethral sphincterotomy
- Augmentation cystoplasty

Consults
- Neurourology

Complications of treatment
- Anticholinergics can cause dry mouth, blurry vision, palpitations, constipation, and urinary retention.
- Alpha blockers can cause hypotension, syncope.
- Stents can migrate and cause urethral injury.
- Sphincterotomy can cause bleeding.
- Dehiscence of anastamosis after augmentation cystoplasty can cause peritonitis.

Prognosis
- Proper planning of bladder management and regular surveillance for persons at risk has led to a drastic decline in mortality and morbidity as a result of reflux and hydronephrosis.
- Renal failure is now an unusual outcome in SCI and deaths from renal causes are few.
- Persons with SCI should be educated early on about the risk for reflux and hydronephrosis and the importance of proactive surveillance measures.

Suggested Readings

Linsenmeyer, TA, Neurogenic bladder following spinal cord injury. In: Kirshblum S, Campagnolo, DI, DeLisa JA, eds. *Spinal Cord Medicine*. Philadelphia: Lippincott Williams & Wilkins; 2002:181–206.

Shingleton WB, Bodner DR. The development of urologic complications in relationship to bladder pressure in spinal cord injured patients. *J Am Paraplegia Soc.* 1993;16(1):14–17.

Bowel Dysfunction: Lower Motor Neuron

Silvia G. Geraci DO ■ Adam B. Stein MD

Description

Injury to the spinal cord involving the conus medullaris or cauda equina often produces an areflexic, or lower motor neuron (LMN), bowel pattern.

Etiology/Types

- Complete LMN pattern
- Incomplete LMN pattern with variable sensation and sphincter control

Epidemiology

- Gastrointestinal (GI) complications are most common among persons over the age of 60 at time of SCI, and those injured >30 years.

Pathogenesis

- Innervation of the external anal sphincter (EAS) via the pudendal nerve is interrupted, resulting in reduced or absent rectal tone.
- Distal colon and rectal dilatation do not stimulate colonic propulsion because of pelvic nerve denervation.
- Myenteric plexus remains intact allowing for continued slow stool propulsion.

Risk Factors

- Neurologic level at or below T12
- Spinal cord infarct

Clinical Features

- Fecal incontinence
- Abdominal distention or discomfort
- Slow colonic transit time

Natural History

- Persons with incomplete injuries will have a greater likelihood of regaining bowel continence.
- Fecal impaction is the most common complication and usually occurs on the left side.
- Incontinent episodes are common because of EAS incompetence and sensory deficits.

Diagnosis

Differential diagnosis

- Spinal shock

- UMN bowel
- Stretch injury to the pudendal nerve
- Diabetic gastroparesis
- Irritable bowel syndrome
- Ileus
- Fecal impaction
- Sphincter abnormalities: infection, tumor, fistulae

History

- Fecal incontinence with abdominal straining (stress pattern)

Exam

- Reduced or absent tone in EAS on rectal exam
- Absent anocutaneous reflex and bulbocavernosus reflex
- Abdominal tenderness and tympani
- Lower extremity sensory motor impairment with diminished deep tendon reflexes

Testing

- Abdominal radiograph can show distension of the colon with stool.
- EMG reveals denervation of the EAS.
- Prolonged rectosigmoid transit times are seen with nuclear medicine transit studies.

Pitfalls

- Practitioners must be able to identify the features of an UMN as compared to a LMN bowel to be able to prescribe an effective treatment regimen.
- Suppositories and rectal stimulation are ineffective means of evacuation because of the absence of an intact reflex arc.

Red Flags

- Rectal bleeding
- Rectal prolapse
- Diarrhea accompanied by fever and other signs of systemic illness

Treatment

Medical

- Water-soluble lubricant
- Bulk laxatives (fiber) as needed to produce well-formed stool

- Postprandial bowel care to take advantage of the gastrocolic reflex
- Abdominal massage
- Digital manual stool removal is an effective means of evacuation
- Tight underwear or shorts to help support pelvic floor and anal sphincter through gluteal adduction

Exercises
- Kegel exercises

Modalities
- Biofeedback for use in incomplete injuries

Surgical
- Colostomy may be considered if unable to achieve satisfactory results by other means.

Consults
- Gastroenterology
- Colorectal surgery

Complications of treatment
- Hemorrhoids, perirectal abscess, and rectal ulcers are common from digital manipulation and straining.

Prognosis
- The goal is to obtain firm, formed stool that can be retained between bowel routines

yet emptied completely with digital evacuation.
- Bowel routines range from postprandial to daily. A predictable scheduled bowel routine will minimize bowel accidents.

Helpful Hints
- Bladder care should be completed prior to bowel routine to prevent vesicoureteral reflux.
- Avoid Valsalva maneuvers outside of bowel care routine to avoid bowel accidents.
- Changes in stool consistency require adjustments in bowel regimen.
- Medication side effects (eg, narcotics and antidepressants) and dietary changes can impact bowel motility and stool consistency.

Suggested Readings

Consortium for spinal cord medicine et al. Neurogenic bowel management in adults with spinal cord injury. *J Spinal Cord Med.* 1998;21(3):248–293.

Luther SL, Nelson AL, Harrow JJ, et al. A comparison of patient outcomes and quality of life in persons with neurogenic bowel: Standard bowel care program vs colostomy. *J Spinal Cord Med.* 2005;28:387–393.

Steins SA, Fajardo NR, Korsten MA. The gastrointestinal system after spinal cord injury. In: Lin VW et al., eds. *Spinal Cord Medicine: Principles and Practice.* New York: Demos; 2003:321–348.

Bowel Dysfunction: Upper Motor Neuron

Silvia G. Geraci DO ■ Adam B. Stein MD

Description
An SCI above the level of the sacral segments produces a bowel pattern characterized by slow colonic propulsion and a competent external anal sphincter (EAS), which favors stool retention.

Etiology/Types
■ Complete UMN pattern
■ Incomplete UMN pattern with variable degree of rectal sensation and EAS control

Epidemiology
■ In one study, 95% of persons with SCI required at least one therapeutic procedure to initiate defecation.
■ It is estimated that 5% to 10% of deaths associated with SCI may result from unidentified GI complications.
■ GI complications are more frequent among persons with cervical and upper thoracic injuries than lower thoracic and lumbosacral injuries.

Pathogenesis
■ Gastrocolic and orthocolic reflexes and myenteric plexus remain intact, allowing for continued slow stool propulsion with segmental peristalsis.
■ The EAS is tonically contracted and competent, though often not under voluntary control.

Risk Factors
■ SCI or disease above the sacral spinal segments

Clinical Features
■ Abdominal bloating
■ Constipation
■ Incontinent episodes

Natural History
■ Uncompensated UMN bowel can lead to significant constipation with or without frequent incontinent episodes.
■ Fecal impaction is the most common complication and is usually right-sided.
■ Chronic severe constipation can lead to nausea/ vomiting, fecal impaction, or megacolon.

Diagnosis

Differential diagnosis
■ Ileus
■ Fecal impaction
■ Intestinal obstruction
■ Volvulus
■ Primary GI carcinoma or metastatic carcinoma to the GI tract
■ Abdominal adhesions

History
■ Delayed evacuation with fecal incontinence
■ Early satiety or loss of appetite
■ Nausea
■ Respiratory compromise if severe abdominal distention

Exam
■ Present anocutaneous reflex (EAS contraction in response to a noxious or tactile stimulation of the perianal skin)
■ Present bulbocavernosus reflex (EAS contraction in response to stimulation of the glans penis or clitoris)
■ Increased EAS tone on digital rectal exam
■ Distended or tender abdomen

Testing
■ Increased colonic transit time on nuclear medicine transit time studies.
■ Intracolonic pressures increase profoundly to small infusion volumes.
■ Intraluminal colonic electromyographic recordings show increased myoelectric activity and dysrhythmic discharges.

Pitfalls
■ Individuals with lesions above T5 may have minimal or no abdominal pain, even with substantial intra-abdominal pathology.
■ Autonomic dysreflexia can be triggered by rectal overdistention, digital rectal stimulation, or perirectal pathology such as abscesses or fistulae.

Red Flags
■ Persistent rectal bleeding or diarrhea
■ Change in a previously stable bowel pattern

- Shortness of breath associated with abdominal distention
- Autonomic dysreflexia during bowel care

Treatment

Medical
- Bowel care is performed at the same time of the day, preferably in sitting position using a commode chair
- Maintain proper balance of fluid intake, diet, and activity to maintain a soft but formed stool consistency
- Water-soluble lubricant (eg, docusate sodium)
- Colonic stimulant (eg, senna, polyethylene glycol)
- Methods of stimulated evacuation include digital stimulation, suppositories, and mini-enemas
- Abdominal massage, push-ups, and leaning forward help to increase intra-abdominal pressures and peristalsis
- A digital stimulator or suppository inserter may be helpful for persons with limited hand function

Modalities
- Pulsed irrigation evacuation

Surgical
- Malone antegrade continence enema
- Colostomy for failure of other bowel management options

Consults
- Gastroenterology
- Surgery, for suspected surgical abdomen

Complications of treatment
- Hemorrhoids, perirectal abcesses, and colocutaneous fistulas may result from chronic manipulation of rectum while performing bowel care.
- Melanosis coli associated with long-term use of senna
- Large-volume enemas can potentially cause autonomic dysreflexia associated with rectal overdistention.

Prognosis
- Goal is to maintain soft-formed stool evacuated in a timely, predictable fashion.
- With a bowel routine performed every 1 to 2 days, episodes of unplanned evacuation were reduced from 64% of bowel movements to 4%.

Helpful Hints
- Ability to transfer, hand dexterity, and caregiver availability must be considered when selecting a bowel routine.
- Safety precautions such as commode seat belts or safety straps should be utilized to prevent falls during bowel care.

Suggested Readings

Consortium for spinal cord medicine et al. Neurogenic bowel management in adults with spinal cord injury. *J Spinal Cord Med.* 1998;21(3):248–293.

Steins SA, Fajardo NR, Korsten MA. The gastrointestinal system after spinal cord injury. In: Lin VW, et al, eds. *Spinal Cord Medicine: Principles and Practice.* New York: Demos; 2003:321–348.

Section I: Conditions

Cardiovascular Issues: Cardiovascular Disease

Kristjan T. Ragnarsson MD

Description

Atherosclerotic disease, primarily affecting coronary arteries, during the chronic phase of SCI.

Etiology/Types

- Sedentary lifestyle and lack of physical exercise
- Impaired exercise capacity due to autonomic dysfunction
- Lipid abnormalities
- Carbohydrate intolerance
- Obesity and proportional increase in body fat

Epidemiology

- Incidence of cardiovascular disease (CVD) rises with duration of SCI and advancing age.
- CVD is the second leading cause of death in patients with SCI.
- CVD is the leading cause of death (46%) of persons with SCI of >30 years duration.
- CVD is the leading cause of death among persons with SCI over 60 years of age (35%).
- Asymptomatic coronary artery disease (CAD) is most common in persons with complete tetraplegia and least common in those with incomplete paraplegia.

Pathogenesis

- Loss of supraspinal control over the sympathetic nervous system following SCI above T6 level results in reduced exercise capacity.
- Paralysis of the largest muscle mass of the body, that is of the lower limbs, is associated with profoundly sedentary lifestyle.
- Reduced exercise capacity and sedentary lifestyle is associated with lipid abnormalities, carbohydrate intolerance, proportionally increased body fat, and obesity, which contribute to arteriosclerosis.

Risk Factors

- High level neurologically complete SCI
- Reduced physical activity
- Low HDL cholesterol
- Impaired glucose intolerance and insulin resistance
- Diabetes mellitus
- Proportional increase in body fat
- Obesity
- Cigarette smoking
- Hypertension
- Psychosocial factors: depression, social isolation, chronic stress

Clinical Features

- Persons with SCI below T6 may have classic symptoms of angina and myocardial infarction (MI). ie, chest and arm pain, and so on.
- Persons with SCI above T6 level may not perceive chest pain but may complain of neck or jaw pain.
- Atypical symptoms of CAD may result in underdiagnosis and delayed treatment.
- Lower limb and/or pulmonary edema may be associated with CAD and congestive heart failure (CHF).

Natural History

- After living for decades with SCI, CVD becomes the most frequent cause of death.

Diagnosis

Differential diagnosis

- Dependent edema versus CAD with CHF
- Atelectasis and pneumonia versus CHF
- Gastroesophageal reflux

History

- Constrictive or crushing pain in chest, shoulders, arms, neck, and/or jaw in persons with SCI below T5
- Absence of chest pain is possible in persons with SCI above T6, who may experience neck, throat, or jaw pain
- Pain relieved by rest or nitroglycerin indicates angina
- Prolonged and more severe pain may indicate MI
- Limb or pulmonary edema
- Excessive perspiration
- Shortness of breath

Exam

- Cardiac murmurs
- High blood pressure
- Edema

Testing

- EKG may reveal characteristic changes for CAD and myocardial infarction (MI)
- Nonspecific ST segment and T-wave changes on EKG may be associated with SCI, rather than CAD
- Chest X-ray
- Arm ergometry stress test cannot be done in persons with tetraplegia
- Consider pharmacologic stress test
- Assess cardiac enzymes

Pitfalls

- Persons with high level SCI may not have classic cardiac pain associated with angina pectoris or MI.

Red Flags

- Chest pain, left shoulder pain, or shortness of breath after minimal activity

Treatment

Medical

- Manage risk factors such as hyperlipidemia, hypertension, and diabetes with appropriate medications,
- Classic vasodilators such as nitroglycerin may not be tolerated due to hypotension
- Aspirin and beta blockers for angina and post-MI
- Use angiotensin-converting enzyme (ACE) inhibitors with caution, if renal insufficiency is present.

Surgical

- Coronary angioplasty or coronary stent insertion
- Coronary artery grafting procedure

Consults

- Cardiology
- Cardiothoracic surgery

Complications of treatment

- Orthostasis with antihypertensives

Prognosis

- Prevention and treatment of risk factors may reduce incidence and prevalence of CAD.
- Effective medical and surgical management of CAD may prevent MI.

Helpful Hints

- Have a high degree of suspicion since CAD is underdiagnosed in persons with SCI.
- Absence of chest pain does not exclude presence of MI, especially in high level SCI.
- Nonspecific EKG changes are common after SCI.

Suggested Readings

Bauman BA, Spungen AM. Coronary heart disease in individuals with spinal cord injury: Assessment of risk factors. *Spinal Cord*. 2008;46:466–476.

Sabharwal S. Cardiovascular dysfunction in spinal cord disorders. In: Lin VW, ed. *Spinal Cord Medicine: Principles and Practice*. New York: Demos; 2003:179–192.

Cardiovascular Issues: Dyslipidemia

Avniel Shetreat-Klein MD PhD

Description

Dyslipidemia is a syndrome of abnormal regulation of lipoproteins. It includes hypertriglyceridemia, hypercholesterolemia, and hyperlipoproteinemia. Elevated serum lipids are a risk factor for coronary artery disease (CAD).

Etiology/Types

- Hyperlipidemia refers to elevated cholesterol and/or triglycerides.
- Hyperlipoproteinemia usually refers to elevated low-density lipoprotein (LDL).
- Combined hyperlipidemia refers to elevated LDL and triglycerides.

Epidemiology

- Inconsistent reports of increased prevalence of dyslipidemia in persons with SCI are found in the literature.
- One study indicates LDL levels were more abnormal in persons with paraplegia than in those with tetraplegia.

Pathogenesis

- Because lipids are insoluble in blood, they must be carried as protein aggregates.
- Dietary triglycerides (fats) and cholesterol enter the bloodstream as *chylomicrons* and are taken up in target tissue.
- Endogenously produced triglycerides (usually in the liver) are carried by very low-density lipoproteins.
- Endogenous cholesterol is carried away from the liver by LDL and is returned to the liver by high-density lipoprotein (HDL).
- Many genetic, hormonal, and metabolic conditions can alter the synthesis and/or metabolism of these lipoproteins and lead to dyslipidemia.

Risk Factors

- Male gender
- Uncontrolled blood sugar
- High carbohydrate (>60% of calories) diet
- Excessive alcohol intake
- History of pancreatitis
- Hypothyroidism
- Nephrotic syndrome
- Decreased activity level

Clinical Features

- Dyslipidemia is typically asymptomatic until secondary complications such as atherosclerosis arise.
- High triglyceride levels can present as abdominal pain or pancreatitis.
- High cholesterol level can present as xanthomas.

Natural History

- Persistent elevations in LDL are associated with increased risk of atherosclerotic disease (CAD, cerebrovascular disease, peripheral vascular disease).

Diagnosis

Differential diagnosis

- Diabetes
- Hypothyroidism

History

- No pathognomonic complaints
- High levels of triglycerides may present as abdominal pain

Exam

- Mild to moderate levels of hyperlipidemia generally lack physical exam abnormalities
- Severe elevation of triglycerides may have abdominal tenderness
- Cutaneous xanthomas
- Ophthalmologic abnormalities (lipid deposition in retina or retinal blood vessels)

Testing

- To distinguish between primary and secondary hyperlipidemia, check glucose, thyroid, and creatinine levels.
- For evaluation of lipids, check fasting levels of: cholesterol, triglycerides, LDL, and HDL.
- Thresholds for treatment depend on pretest CAD risk levels. As persons with SCI are at increased risk for several components of metabolic syndrome, it would be reasonable to treat persons with SCI as intermediate to high risk.
- In general, treat LDL levels >130 mg/dL.
- Target triglyceride levels are <150 mg/dL.

Pitfalls
- Weighing risk factors and evaluating lipid levels to determine treatment can be complex. Referral to internal medicine is prudent for complicated cases.

Red Flags
- Although dyslipidemia may be asymptomatic, the atherosclerosis it can lead to may be deadly. Elevated lipid levels should prompt thorough evaluation of cardiovascular risk levels.

Treatment

Medical
- Dietary and behavior modification
- Low fat diet for overweight persons with high triglycerides
- Omega-3 fatty acids (>10 g/day) have been shown to be effective at lowering triglycerides
- Limit simple carbohydrates and liquid sugars (fruit juices, sodas)
- HMG-CoA reductase inhibitors (statins) to lower elevated LDLs
- Niacin can lower LDL and triglycerides and raise HDL
- Fibric acid derivatives (gemfibrozil, fenofibrate)

Exercises
- Aerobic activity (60 minutes, three times per week)
- Upper extremity ergometry
- Functional electrical stimulation cycle
- Weight loss

Consults
- Internal medicine
- Endocrine
- Cardiology

Complications of treatment
- Statins have well-known complications of myopathy and myalgia.
- In some persons, niacins cause hepatic dysfunction.

Prognosis
- Elevated cholesterol and lipid levels should be correctable with appropriate treatment, lowering risk for cardiovascular disease.

Helpful Hints
- Check cardiovascular risk factors regularly to initiate early treatment

Suggested Readings

Kemp BJ, Spungen AM, Adkins RH, Krause JS, Bauman WA. The relationships among serum lipid levels, adiposity, and depressive symptomatology in persons aging with spinal cord injury. *J Spinal Cord Med*. 2000;23(4):216–220.

Myers J, Lee M, Kiratli J. Cardiovascular disease in spinal cord injury: an overview of prevalence, risk, evaluation, and management. *Am J Phys Med Rehabil*. 2007;86(2):142–152.

Schmidt A, Knoebber J, Vogt S, et al. Lipid profiles of persons with paraplegia and tetraplegia: Sex differences. *J Spinal Cord Med*. 2008;31(3):285–289.

Section I: Conditions

Dysphagia

Dana Spivack David MS CCC-SLP ■ Anne Marie Abdulrauf MA CCC-SLP

Description
Dysphagia is difficulty chewing or swallowing. The entry of any solid or liquid, including saliva, into the trachea is called aspiration.

Etiology/Types
- Oral preparatory phase disorders
- Oral phase disorders
- Oropharyngeal phase disorders
- Pharyngeal phase disorders
- Esophageal swallow disorders

Epidemiology
- Pharyngeal phase disorders account for the vast majority of the dysphagia seen after SCI.

Pathogenesis
- Anterior neck swelling after anterior cervical surgery can lead to reduced laryngeal elevation, poor pharyngeal peristalsis, and reduced epiglottic inversion.
- Injury to the recurrent laryngeal nerve during anterior cervical surgery can lead to vocal fold paralysis.
- Oral intubation can lead to reduced tongue base retraction and/or a laryngeal injury.
- Immobilization of the neck in extension with a cervical orthosis can lead to oral and/or pharyngeal deficits.
- A tracheostomy tube can lead to decreased laryngeal elevation during swallowing.

Risk Factors
- Tracheostomy tube
- Anterior cervical surgery
- Cranial nerve damage
- Traumatic brain injury
- Mechanical ventilation
- Cervical orthoses
- Vocal fold paralysis/paresis

Clinical Features
- Coughing, choking, eye tearing, or frequent throat clearing with eating/drinking
- Wet/gurgly vocal quality with eating/drinking
- Globus sensation in the throat
- Laryngeal penetration; food or liquid goes into the larynx but is cleared before entering the vocal folds, as seen on the modified barium swallow (MBS) study

Natural History
- If dysphagia is left untreated, the patient is at risk for choking, aspiration, and aspiration pneumonia.

Diagnosis

Differential diagnosis
- Reflux
- Esophagitis
- Pharyngitis

History
- Difficulty swallowing food or liquid
- Coughing or choking on food or liquid
- Leaking of food or liquid from mouth
- Pocketing of food in the cheek
- Food stuck in the throat
- History of fevers or pneumonia
- History of swallowing problems

Exam
- On a voluntary cough and swallow without food, a weak cough may suggest poor airway protection or reduced respiratory support
- Reduced lingual/labial range of motion or strength may result in loss of food from mouth, pocketing, or residual of food in cheek/mouth and/or poor propulsion of food to back of mouth
- Coughing, a wet/gurgly vocal quality, frequent throat clearing or choking with swallow trials of various foods (puree to ground/chopped to soft solids to solids) and liquids (thin to nectar-thick to honey-thick liquid) consistency is often indicative of penetration or aspiration
- Reduced initiation or absent swallow
- Decreased laryngeal elevation during swallowing

Testing
- Bedside swallow evaluation
- Blue dye swallow exam
- Modified barium swallow study
- Flexible endoscopic evaluation of swallowing
- Flexible endoscopic evaluation of swallow with sensory testing

Pitfalls
■ Food/liquid trials presented in a controlled environment versus a natural setting (ie, positioning, portion size).

Red Flags
■ Elevated temperature
■ Increased pulmonary congestion
■ Increased oral secretions
■ Increased white blood cell count
■ Pneumonia

Treatment
Medical
■ Diet modifications
■ Reduce rate and amount of intake
■ Alternate swallowing liquids and solids
■ Initiate special swallow techniques (see Exercises)
■ Instruct to turn head when swallowing
■ Position patient upright, as close to 90° as possible
■ Chin-down swallow
■ Nasogastric tube or parenteral feeding if allowed intake is not adequate to meet needs

Exercises
■ Effortful swallow
■ Mendelsohn maneuver
■ Masako maneuver
■ Shaker exercise
■ Supraglottic swallow
■ Super supraglottic swallow
■ Pharyngeal strengthening exercises
■ Oral motor exercises

Modalities
■ Thermal stimulation with ice to the faucial arches
■ Neuromuscular electrical stimulation to the larynx

Injection
■ Vocal fold injection for vocal fold paralysis

Surgical
■ Vocal fold medialization for vocal fold paralysis
■ Percutaneous endoscopic gastrostomy if allowed intake is not adequate to needs

Consults
■ Speech language pathology
■ Otolaryngology
■ Gastroenterology

Complications of treatment
■ Inadequate nutritional intake if prescribed diet is too restrictive
■ Dehydration if not allowed to take liquids or only thickened liquids

Prognosis
■ Good with dysphagia treatment

Helpful Hints
■ The presence of a gag reflex does not ensure a normal swallow.
■ The absence of a gag reflex does not confirm a swallowing disorder.

Suggested Readings
Groher Micheal E. *Dysphagia Diagnosis and Management.* 3rd ed. Newton, MA: Butterworth-Heinemann; 1997.
Logemann Jeri A. *Evaluation and Treatment of Swallowing Disorders.* 2nd ed. Austin, Texas: Pro.ed; 1998.

Section I: Conditions

Endocrine Issues: Glucose Intolerance

Avniel Shetreat-Klein MD PhD

Description
Glucose intolerance is more common in individuals with SCI than in the general population.

Types

Diabetes
- Type 1 diabetes: usually occurs in children and adolescents
- Type 2 diabetes: predominant form of diabetes. Usual onset in middle age

Prediabetes
- Impaired glucose tolerance (IGT): transitional stage en route to diabetes proper. Often undiagnosed
- Fasting hyperglycemia

Epidemiology
- In general, IGT in 11% of population. Diabetes estimated to be in another 6% to 9% of population (including undiagnosed cases)
- In SCI population, 19% with fasting hyperglycemia, 23% to 28% with IGT, and 13% with diabetes
- Level and completeness of injury correlate with degree of impairment in glycemic control
- Persons with SCI become diabetic earlier than those without SCI

Pathogenesis
- The exact sequence of events that leads to diabetes is not fully understood, but, hyperinsulinemia and insulin resistance are found in persons with type 2 diabetes.
- Elevated intramuscular body fat may contribute to glucose intolerance in SCI.
- Hypermetabolic states such as acute trauma can lead to hyperglycemia with increased glucose production.
- Exacerbated in acute phase by high-calorie, high-glycemic index enteral feeds.
- Glucose intolerance can also be caused by infections, and some medications.

Risk Factors
- Type 2 diabetes has genetic influences
- Obesity
- Sedentary lifestyle
- Higher percentage of type 2b muscle fiber (predominates post-SCI)
- Degree of neurologic injury (complete > incomplete)
- Level of injury (tetraplegia > paraplegia)

Clinical Features
- Prediabetes is generally asymptomatic
- Diabetes may have classic features such as thirst, polydipsia, and polyuria, but may be asymptomatic as well
- Abnormal blood sugar (typically elevated, may be abnormally low if on hypoglycemic medication)
- Signs of dehydration and altered mental status in severe cases

Natural History
- Prediabetes can progress to frank diabetes mellitus
- If left untreated can develop multiple complications (see below) including hyperosmolar coma or ketoacidosis
- Increased cardiovascular/cerebrovascular disease risk
- Retinopathy
- Nephropathy
- Neuropathy
- Peripheral vascular disease
- Poor wound healing

Diagnosis

Differential diagnosis
- Type 1 diabetes
- Type 2 diabetes
- Insulin resistance

History
- Excessive thirst, frequent urination
- Visual disturbances
- Neuropathic pain
- Weakness

Exam
- Often normal exam
- May be masked by coexisting deficits from SCI (eg, neuropathic pain, weakness, muscle atrophy)
- Ophthalmologic abnormalities
- Hypertension (frequently associated with glucose intolerance)

Testing

- American Diabetes Association criteria
  - Fasting hyperglycemia = fasting level >100 mg/dL and <126 mg/dL
  - Impaired glucose tolerance = 2-hour oral glucose tolerance test (OGTT) >140 mg/dL and <200 mg/dL
  - Diabetes = fasting level >126 and random glucose >200 mg/dL OR two random glucose levels of >200 mg/dL OR symptoms of diabetes with an abnormal OGTT (>200 mg/dL)
- Urinalysis may show elevated glucose or ketones if severe. Elevated protein may be sign of diabetic nephropathy.
- Glycosylated hemoglobin (Hgb A1c) indicates degree of hyperglycemia in preceding 2 months.
- Metabolic panel
- Lipid testing to assess cardiovascular risk factors

Pitfalls

- Point-of-care testing equipment must be calibrated regularly.
- Use of expired test strips can lead to inaccuracy.

Red Flags

- Severe hypoglycemia can result in coma, seizure, or death.
- Severe hyperglycemia can result in hyperosmolar coma or ketoacidosis.

Treatment

Medical

- In acute SCI, strict glycemic control via subcutaneous (SC) insulin is advisable.
- Long term may need oral hypoglycemics ± SC insulin.

- A well-balanced diet low in fat and total carbohydrates, with an emphasis on low glycemic foods.

Exercises

- Weight loss if appropriate
- Increased physical activity (calorie burning)

Consults

- Internal medicine
- Ophthalmology
- Podiatry
- Endocrine

Complications of treatment

- Overtreatment or mismatch of administered insulin to subsequent food intake can lead to life-threatening hypoglycemia.
- Rapid correction of hyperglycemia alters potassium concentration.

Prognosis

- Strict control can halt progression of complications.

Helpful Hints

- Persons with SCI have below-average fasting glucose, even while showing impaired glucose tolerance.

Suggested Readings

Bauman WA, Adkins RH, Spungen AM, Waters RL. The effect of residual neurological deficit on oral glucose tolerance in persons with chronic spinal cord injury. *Spinal Cord.* 1999;37(11):765–771.

Elder CP, Apple DF, Bickel CS, Meyer RA, Dudley GA. Intramuscular fat and glucose tolerance after spinal cord injury: A cross-sectional study. *Spinal Cord.* 2004;42(12):711–716.

Tharion G, Prasad KR, Gopalan L, Bhattacharji S. Glucose intolerance and dyslipidaemias in persons with paraplegia and tetraplegia in south India. *Spinal Cord.* 1998;36(4):228–230.

Section I: Conditions

Endocrine Issues: Hypercalcemia

Avniel Shetreat-Klein MD PhD

Description
Hypercalcemia is an abnormally high level of calcium ions in the blood stream. It is associated with SCI as a result of immobility-induced increases in bone resorption.

Etiology/Types
- Immobility (decreased weightbearing) results in increased osteoclast-mediated bone resorption, releasing calcium ions.
- Hypercalcemia results when this process exceeds the kidney's ability to excrete calcium.

Epidemiology
- Occurs in 10% to 23% of persons with SCI
- More common in children and people with impaired renal function
- More common in males and those with tetraplegia and complete injuries

Pathogenesis
- The interplay between osteoclast and osteoblast activities responds dynamically to mechanical stress (load) on the bone.
- Piezoelectric forces are thought to play a role.
- Immobility increases osteoclast activity below level of lesion.
- Calcium is then released into the bloodstream, and excreted by kidneys.
- If the kidneys cannot keep up with the calcium efflux (due to renal insufficiency or accelerated bone resorption), hypercalcemia results.
- Secondarily, production of parathyroid hormone is down-regulated, resulting in decreased conversion of vitamin D to its activated form.

Risk Factors
- Immobilization/paralysis
- Renal insufficiency
- Young age (ie, skeletally immature)

Clinical Features
- Typically gradual onset, possibly asymptomatic
- Abnormal lab values generally precede symptoms
- Great variability in clinical presentation may include
  - Mental status changes
  - GI complaints
  - Renal dysfunction
  - Dehydration

Natural History
- Hypercalcemia can occur as early as the first several weeks following acute SCI.
- Bone loss tapers off over time. The risk of hypercalcemia diminishes as the condition becomes chronic.
- Peak period is 4 to 8 weeks postinjury.
- A high index of suspicion is needed for at-risk persons as onset may be insidious.

Diagnosis

Differential diagnosis
- Primary hyperparathyroidism
- Hyperthyroidism
- Acute abdomen
- Constipation
- UTI
- Vitamin D overdose

History
- Recent SCI with prolonged immobilization
- Symptoms can vary widely or be asymptomatic
- Fatigue/lethargy
- Confusion
- Abdominal pain/nausea/vomiting
- Polydipsia/polyuria

Exam
- No specific physical findings

Testing
- Total serum calcium level may underestimate true calcium level in cases of hypoalbuminemia (which is common in SCI)
- Corrected calcium = $[0.8*(4.0-\text{albumin})]$ + measured calcium
- Ionized calcium is a more expensive test, but is more relevant and more accurate
- Parathyroid and 1,25-vitamin D levels can be checked to rule out primary hyperparathyroidism
- Expect low parathyroid hormone levels in hypercalcemia due to immobilization
- Chemistry panel: Electrolytes must be monitored to watch for dehydration or other abnormalities
- Renal ultrasound to check for kidney stones

Pitfalls

- High index of suspicion is needed, as presentation can be highly variable.
- Routine serum calcium can underestimate true (ionized) calcium levels in setting of hypoalbuminemia.

Red Flags

- Renal failure

Treatment

Medical

- Intravenous fluids (with or without furosemide)
- Intravenous pamidronate: single dose may be effective, but may need repeated doses if hypercalcemia recurs
- Oral etidronate has been used in combination with calcitonin
- Monitor electrolytes including phosphate levels when using bisphosphonates

Exercises

- Early mobilization has been shown to decrease hypercalcemia in the non-SCI population.

Consults

- Physical medicine and rehabilitation
- Endocrinology

Complications of treatment

- Intravenous pamidronate use may generate fevers
- Oral bisphosphonates can cause esophageal irritation
- Myalgias

Prognosis

- Generally responds to treatment once initiated

Helpful Hints

- Keep hypercalcemia in mind in the at-risk population (acute SCI, young) as it is best to treat before the person is symptomatic

Suggested Readings

Bauman WA, Spungen AM, Adkins RH, Kemp BJ. Metabolic and endocrine changes in persons aging with spinal cord injury. *Assist Technol.* 1999;11(2):88–96.

Chen B, Mechanick JI, Nierman DM, Stein A. Combined calcitriol-pamidronate therapy for bone hyperresorption in spinal cord injury. *J Spinal Cord Med.* 2001;24(4):235–240.

Gilchrist NL, Frampton CM, Acland RH, et al. Alendronate prevents bone loss in patients with acute spinal cord injury: a randomized, double-blind, placebo-controlled study. *J Clin Endocrinol Metab.* 2007;92(4):1385–1390.

Mechanick JI, Brett EM. Endocrine and metabolic issues in the management of the chronically critically ill patient. *Crit Care Clin.* 2002;18(3):619–641, viii.

Section I: Conditions

Endocrine Issues: Hypogonadism

Avniel Shetreat-Klein MD PhD

Description

Hypogonadism is the decreased production of sex hormones from the ovaries and testes.

Etiology/Types

- Low levels of sex hormones in this population are typically the result of decreased production due to acute stress from trauma, or from dysfunction of the hypothalamic-pituitary axis
- In the general population, primary hypogonadism is much more common than acquired, but this would usually be diagnosed by the time of puberty
- Opioid medications commonly used in SCI may decrease sex hormone levels
- Coexisting brain injury
- Medication side effect (eg, antidepressants, antihypertensives, pain medications)

Epidemiology

- Little data is available on prevalence of hypogonadism in females with SCI
- Prevalence among males with SCI is approximately 50%
- In a study that looked at level of injury, the injuries at T8-T11 were most likely to lead to hormonal abnormalities
- May be more common in acute stage of SCI

Pathogenesis

- Most studies point to abnormalities in the hypothalamic–pituitary axis.
- Levels of gonadotropins leutenizing hormone and follicle stimulating hormone are low as well.
- One theory involves the lack of normal somatic input from below the level of injury to the hypothalamus as the prime cause.
- Another theory centers on imbalance of lean mass and adipose tissue in persons with SCI.
- Increased adipose tissue may decrease levels of gonadotropins.
- Stress and chronic illness can alter cortisol and gonadotropin levels.

Risk Factors

- Risk factors have not been well defined, but extrapolating from the pathophysiology one can infer the following:
  - Recent SCI
  - Chronic stress
  - High adipose to lean fat ratio
  - Use of medications that lower testosterone

Clinical Features

- Lack of energy
- Poor sexual function (multifactorial in SCI)
- Poor concentration/irritability
- Decreased bone density
- Poor wound healing
- Failure to thrive

Natural History

- In some cases hypogonadism presents in the acute phase of SCI and resolves after several months.
- In other cases, may present as chronic

Diagnosis

Differential diagnosis

- Depression
- Primary hypogonadism
- Hypo/hyperthyroidism

History

- Complaints consistent with clinical features described earlier

Exam

- In postpubertal persons, often no physical exam findings
- Gynecomastia
- Muscle atrophy

Testing

- Free testosterone level below 300 ng/dL is abnormal (normal values may vary by institution).
- May check thyroid-stimulating hormone levels to rule out thyroid abnormality.
- Prostate-specific antigen (PSA) levels must be checked before initiating replacement therapy

Pitfalls

- Symptoms of hypogonadism overlap with other common psychological features of SCI.

Red Flags

- Psychological symptoms of hypogonadism may be mistaken for depression, leading to inappropriate treatment with antidepressants, which may further lower testosterone.

Treatment

Medical

- Discontinue medications that may be contributing
- Mainstay of medical treatment is replacement of sex hormone
- Testosterone is available in many preparations
- Intramuscular testosterone (Dose recommendations vary; a recent study used 200 mg/mo. May be given every 2 weeks)
- Transdermal patch: 2.5 to 6 mg/day
- Topical gel: 5 to 10 g of gel applied to upper body daily
- Buccal formulation: 30 mg twice daily

Consults

- Endocrinology

Complications of treatment

- Low sperm count
- Overly frequent or prolonged erections
- Gynecomastia
- Sleep apnea
- Progression of prostate cancer (hence the need to screen PSA level prior to therapy)

Prognosis

- Symptoms generally resolve once treatment is initiated, but long-term treatment may be needed.

Helpful Hints

- Low testosterone is under recognized, and screening should be done for at-risk persons.

Suggested Readings

Clark MJ, Petroski GF, Mazurek MO, et al. Testosterone replacement therapy and motor function in men with spinal cord injury: A retrospective analysis. *Am J Phys Med Rehabil.* 2008;87(4):281–284.

Clark MJ, Schopp LH, Mazurek MO, et al. Testosterone levels among men with spinal cord injury: Relationship between time since injury and laboratory values. *Am J Phys Med Rehabil.* 2008;87(9):758–767.

Kostovski E, Iversen PO, Birkeland K, Torjesen PA, Hjeltnes N. Decreased levels of testosterone and gonadotrophins in men with long-standing tetraplegia. *Spinal Cord.* 2008;46(8):559–564.

Naderi AR, Safarinejad MR. Endocrine profiles and semen quality in spinal cord injured men. *Clin Endocrinol (Oxf).* 2003;58(2):177–184.

Section I: Conditions

Endocrine Issues: Osteoporosis

Kristjan T. Ragnarsson MD ■ Thomas N. Bryce MD

Description
Loss of bone substance occurs in all bones below the neurologic level beginning immediately after SCI.

Etiology
- Weightlessness with bed rest and immobilization
- Vitamin D deficiency
- Metabolic factors related to SCI

Epidemiology
- All persons with SCI are affected
- Appears to be more profound in those with neurologically complete SCI

Pathogenesis
- Immobilization results in increased osteoclastic activity.
- Osteoclastic activity results in relative hypercalcemia and hypercalciuria.
- Hypercalcemia inhibits PTH production.
- This secondary hypoparathyroidism inhibits the conversion of the storage form of vitamin D, 25-OH vitamin D to the active form of vitamin D, 1,25-OH vitamin D.
- Bone mineral density (BMD) loss is greatest in distal femur and proximal tibia.
- Trabecular bone is affected first, followed by cortical bone.

Risk Factors
- Paralysis, especially flaccid and neurologically complete
- Immobilization and weightlessness

Clinical Features
- Hypercalcemia and hypercalciuria during acute SCI, especially severe in adolescents
- Usually asymptomatic
- Pathologic fractures

Natural History
- The greatest loss of BMD occurs during the first 4 months after SCI (1% to 2% per week).
- Significant loss of BMD continues for the next 12 months (0.5% to 1% per month).
- Continuous lifelong loss of BMD is estimated to be 0.1% to 1% per year.
- Most women with complete SCI and most men with complete tetraplegia will reach a fracture threshold (the level of BMD below which most fractures occur) at the knee within a few years after injury and then progress to a fracture breakpoint (the level of BMD where the majority of fractures occur).
- Most men with complete paraplegia may reach a fracture threshold without reaching a fracture breakpoint.

Diagnosis

Differential diagnosis
- Primary hypoparathyroidism
- Familial osteoporosis
- Vitamin D deficiency

History
- Prior long bone or compression spinal fractures after minimal or no trauma

Exam
- Kyphotic posture
- Evidence of prior pathologic fractures

Testing
- Radiological studies show osteopenia.
- Dual energy X-ray absorptiometry is the gold standard for diagnosing osteoporosis.
- Quantitative CT is also useful for diagnosing osteoporosis.
- Low serum vitamin D levels predispose to osteoporosis.
- Low serum PTH indicates secondary hypoparathyroidism.
- Serum calcium is often elevated in adolescents, especially boys.

Pitfalls
- Failure to diagnose vitamin D deficiency
- Failure to diagnose osteoporosis

Red Flags
- Vitamin D deficiency
- Long bone fractures with minimal trauma

Treatment

Medical

- Calcium supplementation (daily intake at least 1500 mg) for everyone
- Vitamin D supplementation (daily intake at least 1000 IU) for everyone
- Strongly consider empirical use of a bisphosphonate (pamidronate, alendronate, ibandronate, zoledronate, etc.) in all women with complete SCI and in all men with complete tetraplegia.
- Consider empirical use of a bisphosphonate in all men with complete paraplegia especially if they are physically active and at increased risk for trauma.
- Treat others with bisphosphonates depending on results of quantitative diagnostic testing.

Exercises

- Use of a tilt table or standing frame for those unable to stand
- Standing and ambulating

Modalities

- Functional electrical stimulation (FES) ergometry or ambulation
- Ultrasonic stimulation

Consults

- Endocrinology

Complications of treatment

- Osteonecrosis of jaw with bisphosphonates
- Hyperphosphatemia with bisphosphonates
- Esophagitis with bisphosphonates
- Fracture of long bones from FES ergometry or weight-bearing in those with osteoporosis

Prognosis

- The effectiveness of current preventive and therapeutic interventions is modest.

Helpful Hints

- Early mobilization with weight bearing after injury may help decrease initial rate of bone loss.
- It is never too late to start treatment.

Suggested Readings

Bauman WA, Spungen AM. Endocrinology and metabolism. In: Kirshblum S, Campanolo DL, LeLisa JA, eds. *Spinal Cord Medicine*. Philadelphia: Lippincott Williams & Wilkins; 2002:164–180.

Garland DE, Adkins RH, Stewart CA. Five-year longitudinal bone evaluations in individuals with chronic complete spinal cord injury. *J Spinal Cord Med*. 2008;31(5): 543–50.

Kiratli BJ: Bone loss in osteoporosis following spinal cord injury. In: Lin VW, ed. *Spinal Cord Medicine. Principles and Practice*. New York: Demos; 2003:539–548.

Section I: Conditions

Geriatric Spinal Cord Injury

Kristjan T. Ragnarsson MD

Description
Geriatric SCIs include persons over the age of 60 years with SCI.

Etiology/Types
- Acute SCI in persons over the age of 60
- Persons who sustain SCI earlier in their lives and live past the age of 60

Epidemiology
- Falls (60%)
- Motor vehicle crashes (30%)
- Rising incidence as the population ages
- A 4.5% of all traumatic SCI during the 1970s
- A 11.5% of all traumatic SCI during the 1990s
- Nontraumatic SCI, such as due to disease in the elderly, is more common than traumatic SCI.
- Gender difference is less striking than in younger population.

Pathogenesis
- Major trauma with neurologically complete SCI
- Minor trauma in presence of narrow cervical spinal canal (cervical spinal stenosis) when injury occurs at later age usually resulting in incomplete SCI
- Central cord syndrome is relatively common.

Risk Factors
- Impaired balance and cognition
- Unsafe environment
- Cervical spinal stenosis
- Automobile headrests providing insufficient protection

Clinical Features
- Neurological impairment associated with SCI
- History of cervical spondylosis
- Higher rates of medical complications
- Higher prevalence of preexisting medical conditions
- Slower progress toward functional goals
- Shorter rehabilitation length of stay
- More often discharged to nursing homes

Natural History
- Functional decline occurs earlier.
- Aging process may be hastened by SCI.

- Health is adversely affected by advancing age, duration of SCI, and severity of neurological impairment.
- Conditions more common in older persons with SCI include heart disease, diabetes mellitus, lipid abnormalities, urolithiasis, bladder cancer, bowel irregularities, pressure ulcers, and pneumonia.

Diagnosis
Differential diagnosis
- Nontraumatic causes for SCI
- Variety of acquired neurological conditions

History
- Trauma, major or minor
- Preexisting cervical spondylosis

Exam
- Perform general physical and neurologic examination, including an ASIA motor and sensory examination.
- Assess and observe for comorbidities.

Testing
- Imaging studies may reveal spondylosis and spinal stenosis, but no fracture or dislocation.
- MRI may show abnormal cord signals correlating with the severity of neurological impairment.
- Laboratory tests appropriate for suspected or confirmed comorbidities

Pitfalls
- Underestimating risk of comorbidities
- Overestimating functional goals

Red Flags
- Decline in neurologic function
- Delirium
- Respiratory insufficiency

Treatment
Medical
- Acute SCI: Consider high dose methylprednisolone
- Aggressive prophylaxis for potential comorbidities and treatment when they exist
- Orthoses and assistive equipment as indicated by functional impairment
- High technology devices for those with tetraplegia

Exercises

- Strengthening of innervated muscles
- Range of motion exercises for paralyzed limbs
- Training in activities of daily living (ADLs), ambulation, and wheelchair mobility

Surgical

- Early decompression and/or spinal stabilization as clinically indicated
- Role of surgery is controversial in absence of fracture, dislocation, and/or severe spinal stenosis.

Consults

- Physical medicine and rehabilitation
- Spinal surgery
- Neurourology
- Internal medicine and its subspecialties as clinically indicated
- Geriatrics
- Plastic surgery for pressure ulcers

Complications of treatment

- Failure of surgical fixation due to osteoporotic bone
- Skin breakdown under orthoses

Prognosis

- Higher rates of medical complications following acute SCI than in younger individuals
- Lower levels of independence in ADL and mobility are reached than in younger individuals.

Helpful Hints

- In teaching new techniques, try to mimic what the person has been doing their entire life. For example, teaching a squat pivot transfer to someone with an incomplete SCI may be more successful than teaching a sliding board transfer.
- Consider power mobility for all primary geriatric wheelchair users if environment will support one.

Suggested Readings

Charlifue S. Effect of Aging on Individuals with Chronic SCI. *Topics in SCI Rehabilitation.* 2007;12:3.

Kemp B, Adams RH. Aging with Spinal Cord Injury. *Topics in SCI Rehabilitation.* 2001;6:3.

Whitenek G, Charlifue S, Gerhart KA, et al., eds. *Aging with Spinal Cord Injury.* New York: Demos, 1993.

Section I: Conditions

Mononeuropathies

Youssef Josephson DO

Description
In persons with SCI, the upper limbs are subject to increased pressures and overuse as they become the primary means of weight bearing, locomotion, and transfers. This stress can lead to compressive peripheral nerve injuries or compression mononeuropathies (CMN).

Etiology/Types

Carpal tunnel syndrome
- The most commonly described CMN
- The median nerve is compressed as it passes through the carpal tunnel.
- Cross-sectional studies found a prevalence of 40% to 66% in people with SCI.

Ulnar nerve entrapment at Guyon's canal in the wrist
- Most common in persons with paraplegia using axillary crutches with horizontal palm bars

Ulnar nerve entrapment at the elbow
- Typically resulting from armrest pressure

Radial nerve compression
- Associated with humeral fractures (Holstein-Lewis fracture)

Epidemiology
- More common in persons with paraplegia
- More common in persons using manual wheelchairs
- More common in men

Pathogenesis
- Nerve injury occurs secondary to compression or traction as the nerve passes between muscles, ligaments, or bone.
- Influenced by systemic disorders, obesity, and pregnancy
- Repetitive injury and trauma to a nerve results in microvascular (ischemic) changes and edema, leading to injury and structural changes of both the myelin sheath and axon proper.
- Overuse can occur from repetitive limb tasks or increased force during tasks.

Risk Factors
- Repetitive mechanical loading
- Obesity
- Manual wheelchair use
- Uneven (uphill) transfers
- Improper ergonomics during work or ADLs

Clinical Features
- Progressive pain at the wrist or elbow
- Parathesias
- Progressive weakness and atrophy
- Loss of function

Natural History
- Sensory changes are usually first to occur with parathesias in a peripheral nerve distribution
- Progressive increases in aching pain with continued compression or overuse
- Eventual weakness and muscle atrophy
- Permanent pain and dysfunction if untreated

Diagnosis

Differential diagnosis
- Tendonitis
- Tenosynovitis
- Arthritis
- Vitamin B_{12} deficiency
- Nerve root compression
- Brachial plexopathy
- Syringomyelia

History
- Painful parathesias ("pins and needles") that are worse at night
- Usually unilateral
- Worsening of aching pain in hands or elbows
- Clumsiness during ADLs

Exam
- Tinel's sign at suspected site of compression
- Altered sensation over the sensory nerve distribution
- Weakness or atrophy in muscles innervated by the respective nerve

Testing
- Nerve conduction studies will show a significant drop in conduction velocity or amplitude across the compression site.

- EMG will display signs of denervation in affected muscles if axonal damage has occurred.
- If clinically indicated, MRI can be used to rule out a mass causing nerve compression.
- Diagnostic nerve block injections may be helpful in confirming a diagnosis.
- A normal HbA1C or TSH can rule out specific metabolic causes.

Red Flags

- Finding multiple neuropathies may be a sign of a systemic problem such as metabolic or vascular abnormalities rather than focal nerve compressions.

Treatment

Medical

- Nonsteroidal anti-inflammatory medications
- Neuromodulatory agents (eg, gabapentin)
- Corticosteroid injections
- Weight loss
- Splinting
- Padded gloves

Exercises

- Proper ergonomic training to prevent further injury
- Optimize manual wheelchair propulsion by promoting lower stroke frequency.
  - Less wheel strokes to achieve the desired speed
- Transfer "downhill"
- Avoidance of extreme wrist positions

Modalities

- Heat/ice
- Transcutaneous electrical nerve stimulation
- Ultrasound

Surgical

- Surgery is indicated with progression of symptoms despite conservative measures.

Consults

- Physical medicine and rehabilitation or neurology for electrodiagnostic testing
- Physical medicine and rehabilitation for treatment
- Hand surgery

Complications of treatment

- Side effects vary by medication
  - NSAIDs: GI irritation, bleeding risk
  - Gabapentin: peripheral edema, psychiatric manifestations at high doses
  - Surgery: additional nerve damage, bleeding, infection, scar formation with limitation of range of motion

Prognosis

- Relief of compression by activity modification or surgery can halt progression of nerve damage.
- Recovery is variable, depending on degree of injury.

Helpful Hints

- Be vigilant to address the issues of upper-extremity pain with each follow-up visit.
- Check that individuals perform daily activities (wheelchair mobility, transfers) with joint protection in mind.

Suggested Reading

Paralyzed Veterans of America Consortium for Spinal Cord Medicine. Preservation of upper limb function following spinal cord injury: A clinical practice guideline for health-care professionals. *J Spinal Cord Med.* 2005;28(5):434–470.

Section I: Conditions

Musculoskeletal Issues: Back Pain

Igor Rakovchik DO ■ Thomas N. Bryce MD

Description
Persons with SCI, particularly those who are ambulatory and have spasticity or weakness that causes gait deviations, often develop chronic musculoskeletal back pain.

Etiology/Types
- Myofascial (muscle strain)
- Facet joint
- Sacroiliac (SI) joint
- Discogenic

Epidemiology
- The back is the most common location of chronic pain after SCI.

Pathogenesis
- Repetitive extension of the spine loads the facet joints and leads to degeneration and pain over time.
- Mobile vertebrae adjacent to fused vertebrae degenerate more quickly.
- Muscle imbalances due to weakness of the dynamic hip stabilizers and/or spasticity during ambulation lead to increased SI joint torsional stresses.
- Repetitive SI joint torsional stresses lead to SI joint degeneration and pain over time.
- Hip hiking is a common gait deviation, which can stress the SI joint.
- Since the outer one-third of the disk annulus is innervated, a tear of the annulus can cause inflammatory substances to leak out of the nucleus pulposis, irritating the now exposed nerve fibers causing discogenic pain.

Clinical Features
- Aggravated by movement
- Relieved by rest

Natural History
- Chronic muscle strains typically will progress unless the precipitating overuse is addressed.
- Degenerative processes of the facet or SI joints that cause pain are typically progressive if exacerbating factors are not addressed, ie, muscle imbalance affecting gait.

Diagnosis

Differential diagnosis
- Spinal instrumentation breakage or failure
- Radicular pain
- At level spinal cord pain
- Below level spinal cord pain
- Charcot spine
- Vertebral fracture

History
- Dull and achy pain located just lateral to the sacrum and worse with extension often indicates SI joint pain.
- Slowly progressive pain located just lateral to the spine worse with extension can indicate facet joint pain.
- Persistent pain worse with flexion and sitting and better with standing and walking can indicate discogenic pain.

Exam
- Myofascial pain
  - Painful trigger points
- Facet pain
  - Pain triggered by spinal extension and rotation
  - Pain relief with flexion
  - Point tenderness just lateral to posterior midline
  - Tight hamstrings
- Sacroilitis
  - Tenderness over the SI joint
  - Positive flexion abduction external rotation (FABER) test
- Discogenic pain
  - Pain triggered by spinal flexion

Testing
- A fluoroscopically guided (FG) SI joint injection for SI joint pain
- X-rays and MRI may reveal facet arthropathy.
- Medial branch nerve blocks or intra-articular facet joint injections for facet joint pain
- Provocative lumbar discography for discogenic pain

Pitfalls
- Be aware that a compressed nerve or root can be the source of muscle pain.

Red Flags
- New neurologic deficits or spinal deformity

Treatment

Medical
- Avoidance of activities that reproduce the pain as much as possible
- Topical or oral nonsteroidal anti-inflammatory drugs (NSAIDs)
- Topical local anesthetic patches
- Evaluation of wheelchair and seating system

Exercises
- Myofascial release for myofascial pain
- Spinal stabilization exercises with a flexion bias for facet joint pain
- Postural re-education to reduce the lordotic curve for facet joint pain
- Lumbo-pelvic stabilization exercises with a flexion bias for SI joint pain
- Gait training to eliminate gait deviations
- Strengthen weak musculature
- Spinal stabilization exercises with an extension bias for discogenic pain

Modalities
- Ice
- Heat (not for areas with impaired sensation due to the risk of burns)
- Electrical stimulation

Injection
- FG medial branch nerve ablations or FG intra-articular facet joint injections for facet joint pain
- FG SI joint injections for SI joint pain
- Local trigger point injections for myofascial pain

Surgical
- Spinal fusion for unrelieved discogenic or facet joint pain

Consults
- Physical medicine and rehabilitation
- Spine surgery
- Interventional pain medicine

Complications of treatment
- Infection, bleeding, nerve injury from interventional and surgical procedures
- Gastrointestinal and renal complications from NSAIDs
- Burns from heating modalities

Prognosis
- Poor if the exacerbating factors are not addressed, ie, muscle imbalance affecting gait.

Suggested Readings

Cooper G, Herrera JE, Dambeck M. Lower back injuries. In: Herrera JE, Cooper G, eds. *Essential Sports Medicine*. Totowa: Humana, 2008: 99–114.

Irwin RW, Restrepo JA, Sherman A. Musculoskeletal pain in persons with spinal cord injury. *Top Spinal Cord Inj Rehabil*. 2007;13(2):43–57.

Section I: Conditions

Musculoskeletal Issues: Contracture

Anousheh Behnegar MD ■ Thomas N. Bryce MD

Description

Contracture is a limitation in joint range of motion (ROM).

Etiology/Types

- Bony
- Tendinous/ligamentous
- Intrinsic muscle
- Spastic muscle

Epidemiology

- Occurs after 5% to 10% of SCI
- More common in persons with tetraplegia
- More common in persons with complete injury
- Twice as common in those with spasticity (13% vs 8%)
- Twice as common in those with pressure ulcers (14% vs 7%)

Pathogenesis

Bony

- Heterotopic ossification (HO)
- Activation of pluripotential mesenchymal cells in the soft tissue to switch their differentiation from fibro-progenitor to osteoprogenitor pathway
- Local production of bone morphogenic protein (BMP)

Tendonous/ligamentous

- Fibrosis, hyalinization, and fibrinoid degeneration

Intrinsic muscle

- Shortening of muscle fibers
- Intramuscular fibrosis
- Hastened by spasticity

Spastic muscle

- Loss of inhibitory control of the alpha- and gamma motoneurons

Risk Factors

- Tetraplegia
- Traumatic brain injury
- Joint immobilization
- Joint pain
- Delayed rehabilitation

Clinical Features

- Loss of ROM of any joint, especially in those joints with active movement in only one direction
- Loss of elbow extension ROM in those with a C5 or C6 neurologic level
- Loss of hip extension ROM in those with L1–L5 neurologic levels
- Loss of ankle dorsiflexion ROM in those with pre-served plantar flexion strength as compared to ankle dorsiflexion strength

Natural History

- Loss of ROM is usually initially reversible.
- The longer a joint remains unmoved, the more likely permanent changes will take place.
- Loss of joint ROM leads to loss of limb function.

Diagnosis

Differential diagnosis

- Pain limiting joint ROM
- Fractures

History

- Prolonged joint immobilization
- Severe spasticity
- Insidious onset of loss of joint ROM

Exam

- Hard endpoint to diminished passive ROM indicates either tendinous/ligamentous or bony contracture.
- Soft endpoint to diminished passive ROM indicates either intrinsic muscle contracture or spastic muscle-related contracture.
- Loss of internal and external rotation at the hips is commonly seen before a limitation in flexion for bony contracture related to HO.

Testing

- Joint X-rays
- Triple-phase bone scan to evaluate for noncalcified HO
- ROM under anesthesia may eliminate the contributing factors of pain and spasticity.

Pitfalls

- Bony, tendinous/ligamentous, intrinsic muscle, and spastic muscle contracture can all coexist.

Red Flags
- Joint that is ankylosed

Treatment

Medical
- Antispasticity medications (baclofen, tizanidine, benzodiazepines) can treat spasticity.
- Dynamic splinting and serial casting
- Bisphosphonates and NSAIDs can treat noncalcified HO.

Exercise
- Stretching and ROM exercises are the mainstays of treatment, but are most successful in treating spastic muscle-related contracture.

Modalities
- Ice can diminish spasticity.
- Heat can facilitate stretching.

Injection
- Neurotoxin or alcohol/phenol injections can reduce spasticity.

Surgical
- Tenotomy and tendon-lengthening procedures
- Wedge or bone resection
- Intrathecal pump insertion for baclofen administration

Consults
- Physical medicine and rehabilitation
- Orthopedic surgery

Complications of treatment
- Long bone fractures from aggressive ROM
- Altered biomechanics due to tendon lengthening
- Excessive blood loss and poor wound healing after bone resection
- Contracture recurrence

Prognosis
- Once tendinous/ligamentous contracture has developed, the prognosis for nonsurgical reversal is poor.
- Antispasticity medication is usually successful in treating spastic muscle-related contracture.

Helpful Hints
- Regular and early ROM beginning in the intensive care setting can limit the effects of spasticity and prevent tendinous/ligamentous contracture from developing.
- Teach family members how to do joint ROM early as ROM by staff is all to often neglected due to other more acute medical needs taking precedence.
- Early implantation of an intrathecal baclofen pump may limit the ultimate development of muscular and tendinous/ligamentous contracture.

Suggested Reading
Dalyan D, Sherman A, Cardenas DD. Factors associated with contractures in acute spinal cord injury. *Spinal Cord.* 1998;36:405–408.

Section I: Conditions

Musculoskeletal Issues:
Heterotopic Ossification

Igor Rakovchik DO ■ Thomas N. Bryce MD

Description
Heterotopic ossification (HO) is true bone formation at ectopic sites outside the skeleton, most frequently around a joint.

Etiology/Types
- Brookers X-ray classification:
  - Class 1: isolated bone islands
  - Class 2: >1 cm between opposing ossification centers
  - Class 3: <1 cm between opposing ossification centers
  - Class 4: joint ankylosis

Epidemiology
- The hip is by far the most common site of development after SCI, followed by the knee, shoulder, and elbow.
- Onset is usually 1 to 4 months postinjury
- Occurs in 40% to 50% of the adult population with SCI
- 0% to 20% have significant limitation in ROM
- 5% progress to ankylosis
- HO usually reaches maturity within 1.5 to 2 years
- Occurs below the level of neurological injury

Pathogenesis
- Thought to be due to a general inflammatory response following injury that causes release of inflammatory cytokines, which trigger pluripotential mesenchymal stem cells in soft tissues to differentiate into osteoblasts.
- These osteoblasts form an extracellular matrix (osteoid) within the soft tissue.
- The osteoid matrix is mineralized by deposition of crystalline hydroxyapatite.
- Osteoblasts and osteoclasts couple to remodel the bone under the control of various hormones, vitamin D metabolites, prostaglandins, and growth factors to form mature HO.

Risk Factors
- Complete SCI
- Spasticity
- Pressure ulcers
- Extremity trauma

Clinical Features
- Localized tissue swelling
- Decreased joint ROM

Natural History
- Bone growth begins in the periphery and grows inward to the central part of the lesion.
- Progression is variable.

Diagnosis

Differential diagnosis
- Deep vein thrombosis
- Fracture
- Septic joint
- Tumor

History
- Inability to lean forward in the wheelchair or reach feet
- Pain with ROM of the affected joint
- Leg swelling

Exam
- Periarticular localized tissue swelling
- Decreased joint ROM
- Joint effusion
- Low-grade fever

Testing
- A triple-phase bone scan is the current gold standard for early detection of HO (before changes appear on X-ray).
- X-rays only pick up HO when there is evidence of calcification present.
- Bone scans normalize after 6 to 18 months as HO matures and is no longer active.
- Serum alkaline phosphatase increases at 2 weeks, exceeds normal at 3 weeks, peaks at 10 weeks, and returns to normal after HO matures.

Pitfalls
- Pharmacologic interventions have not shown great effectiveness if started when there is already evidence of HO on X-ray.

Red Flags

- HO that grows around the joints such as the knees and elbows may compress neurovascular structures, such as the popliteal artery or ulnar nerve, respectively.

Treatment

Medical

- Etidronate disodium (Didronel) (20 mg/kg/day by mouth for 6 months)
- Indomethacin or other NSAIDs
- Medications are typically only effective when treatment is started before there is evidence of mature heterotopic bone on X-ray.
- Low-dose radiation has been reported to control HO and avoid recurrence following surgery. It is given in a single fraction either just before or right after surgery.

Exercises

- ROM exercises avoiding excessive force and muscle trauma

Surgical

- The primary goal for removal of HO is to promote easier positioning, transfers, and ADLs.
- Wheelchair seating may be the only indication for resection.
- Surgery should only be attempted when HO is mature and the bone scan and alkaline phosphatase are normal.
- Wedge resection is the most common type of surgical excision.

Consults

- Physical medicine and rehabilitation
- Orthopedic surgery
- Radiation oncology

Complications of treatment

- Forcible stretching can cause clinical or microscopic hemorrhage, which can lead to new HO formation.
- Some persons may develop hyperphosphatemia from use of etidronate.
- Infection and neurovascular injury can occur after surgery.
- Recurrence of HO is common after surgery.

Prognosis

- Only a small minority of persons with HO require surgical intervention and generally HO is self-limited.

Helpful Hints

- A reevaluation of wheelchair seating including pressure mapping should be performed if there is significant loss of joint ROM in order to minimize skin breakdown and discomfort from a poorly fitting wheelchair.

Suggested Readings

Banovac K, Gonzalez PA, Renfree, KJ. Treatment of heterotopic ossification after spinal cord injury. *J Spinal Cord Med.* 1997;20:60–65.

Montroy R. Heterotopic ossification. In Lin V, ed. *Spinal Cord Medicine: Principles and Practice.* New York: Demos; 2003:613–622.

Section I: Conditions

Musculoskeletal Issues: Osteoporotic Limb Fractures

Kristjan T. Ragnarsson MD ■ Thomas N. Bryce MD

Description
Osteoporotic bones in chronically paralyzed limbs can fracture with minimal trauma.

Etiology/Types
- Trauma, often minor, eg, a fall during transfer or excessive stretching of a paralyzed limb
- Spontaneous, ie, no recognized trauma

Epidemiology
- Exact annual incidence is unknown.
- Less than 10% of persons with chronic SCI report having had limb fractures.
- The fracture rate is 10 times greater in those with complete injuries as compared to those with incomplete injuries.
- Fractures may go unnoticed in paralyzed anesthetic limbs.

Pathogenesis
- Bone loss is greatest in distal femur and proximal tibia where fractures are most common.

Risk Factors
- Osteoporosis
- Trauma
- Neurologically complete SCI with flaccid paralysis
- People with paraplegia are more prone to fractures than those with tetraplegia.

Clinical Features
- Painless swelling and/or deformity
- Most common around the knee
- Pathologic spine and hip fractures are rare.

Natural History
- If the long bone fracture is adequately immobilized and not significantly displaced, healing should occur within several weeks with exuberant callus.
- Shortening of the limb and angular deformities are common and can often be prevented with open reduction and internal fixation.

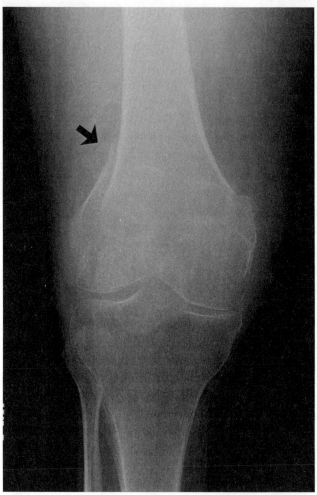

Fracture of the supracondylar region of the femur (arrow).

Diagnosis

Differential diagnosis
- Deep vein thrombosis
- Heterotopic ossification
- Infection/cellulitis
- Contusion
- Arthritis

History
- Often noncontributory
- Trauma, often insignificant

- Increased spasticity
- Increased autonomic symptoms, eg, sweating and lightheadedness

Exam
- Knee swelling with increased intra-articular fluid
- Bony instability
- Local crepitations, palpable or audible

Testing
- X-rays
- CT scan
- Isotope bone scan

Pitfalls
- Absence of pain does not exclude fracture.
- Initial X-rays may not show a hairline fracture.

Red Flags
- Open fracture
- Severe angulation
- Rotational deformity

Treatment

Medical
- Treatment goals: prevent complications and preserve function.
- Traditional fracture management is indicated for ambulatory persons who have neurologically incomplete SCI.
- A nonsurgical approach is preferred for nonambulatory persons with neurologically complete SCI and a nondisplaced or minimally displaced lower extremity fracture.
- Distal femur and proximal tibia fractures are typically minimally displaced and are best treated with a well-padded splint or knee immobilizer.
- Slight shortening and angulation of bone is acceptable.
- Rotational deformity is unacceptable as it may result in suboptimal foot placement on the wheelchair's footrest.

- Circular casts are best avoided, but if applied, must be bivalved to permit regular skin inspection.
- Permit wheelchair mobility early.

Surgical
- A displaced femoral neck fracture is best treated with a prosthesis replacement; if left untreated the femur can migrate proximally, unbalancing the pelvis.
- A displaced intertrochanteric fracture is best treated with an intramedullary hip fixation device in order to prevent varus hip deformity.
- A displaced femoral shaft fracture is best treated with an interlocking intramedullary rod.
- A displaced tibial shaft fracture is best treated with an interlocking intramedullary nail.

Consults
- Orthopedic surgery

Complications of treatment
- Skin breakdown from immobilizing cast or brace
- Subluxation and dislocation of femoral prosthesis used for femoral neck fracture
- External fixation predisposes to trophic ulcers

Prognosis
- Most fractures heal well in 3 to 8 weeks, often with exuberant callus formation.
- Nonunion is rare and is relatively insignificant clinically in non–weight-bearing limbs.

Helpful Hints
- Have a high degree of suspicion, especially for unexplained knee swelling
- Avoid surgical interventions in neurologically complete SCI.
- Prevent rotational deformities but accept some shortening and angulation.

Suggested Reading
Garland D, Shokes L. Management of long bone fractures.
In: Lin VW, ed. *Spinal Cord Medicine, Principles and Practice.*
New York: Demos; 2003:535–538.

Section I: Conditions

Musculoskeletal Issues: Shoulder Pain

Igor Rakovchik DO ■ Thomas N. Bryce MD

Description
Shoulder pain after SCI is typically musculoskeletal and the result of overuse from wheelchair propulsion, transfers, and other ADLs.

Etiology/Types
- Rotator cuff impingement syndrome
  - Subacromial bursitis
  - Bicipital tendonitis
  - Supraspinatus tendonitis
- Glenohumeral instability
- Adhesive capsulitis
- Osteoarthritis

Epidemiology
- The most common painful joint
- Prevalence 40% to 60% overall
- Prevalence may be greater early after tetraplegia
- Prevalence increases over time after paraplegia
- Interferes with self-care in 30% to 50%

Pathogenesis

Rotator cuff impingement syndrome
- Overuse of the shoulders can lead to glenohumeral ligament and labrum microtrauma with resultant mild glenohumeral instability.
- The rotator cuff or the dynamic shoulder stabilizers compensate and become fatigued.
- The humeral head is allowed to migrate upward impinging the rotator cuff against the coracoacromial arch, causing pain.
- This process is hastened by
  - Rotator cuff and scapular stabilizer muscle imbalance due to unbalanced repetitive upper extremity activity (transfers, wheelchair propulsion, etc.)
  - Rotator cuff and scapular stabilizer muscle weakness due to cervical SCI
  - Rotator cuff tears from repeated impingement.

Osteoarthritis
- Repetitive use over time
- Exacerbated by glenohumeral instability

Risk Factors
- Use of a manual wheelchair
- Overhead activities
- Greater body mass index
- Increased duration of injury
- Poor seated posture
- Limited shoulder girdle flexibility
- Older age
- Female gender

Clinical Features
- Pain with ROM
- Pain when weightbearing through the shoulders
- Pain with ADLs and transfers

Natural History
- Worsening pain
- Decreased functional mobility including the loss of the ability to transfer and propel a manual wheelchair

Diagnosis

Differential diagnosis
- Cervical radiculopathy
- Syrinx causing pain
- Myofascial pain

History
- Painful shoulder ROM
- Pain when sitting in chair or lying on shoulder

Exam
- Neer and Hawkin's test for impingement
- Apprehension, relocation, load shift tests for capsular instability
- Yergason's and Speed's tests for bicipital tendonitis
- Sulcus sign for ligamentous laxity
- Drop-arm test for rotator cuff tear
- Cross-arm test for acromioclavicular arthrosis

Testing
- Plain radiographs
- EMG/nerve conduction studies
- MRI/CT

Pitfalls
- May be very difficult to differentiate from other pain syndromes
- More than one pain generator may be present at any one time.

Red Flags

- Loss of ROM
- New weakness not due to pain
- Associated sensory loss or changes over the shoulder can indicate neurologic cause.

Treatment

Medical

- NSAIDs
- If the dynamic shoulder stabilizers are unable to maintain glenohumeral positioning, ensure adequate arm support in the wheelchair and bed.
- Minimize transfers.
- Vary the direction of transfers.
- Avoid uneven surface transfers.
- Avoid raising hand above the shoulder.
- Avoid end range positions of the shoulder.
- Use the lightest possible manual wheelchair.
- Facilitate weight loss if overweight.
- Instruct in proper wheelchair propulsion technique.
- Ensure optimal positioning in the wheelchair.
- If pain is chronic, strongly consider use of a power wheelchair.

Exercises

- A balanced shoulder-strengthening program is the mainstay of treatment.
- A stretching program to maintain flexibility of the shoulder girdle
- Postural retraining

Modalities

- Heat
- Cold
- Ultrasound
- Electrical stimulation for strengthening weak muscles

Injection

- Intra-articular steroid injections: limit to three per lifetime for the glenohumeral joint
- Intra-articular hyalgan injections
- Peritendonous sheath injections

Surgical

- Recurring dislocations, tendonitis, and severe arthritis may require surgery.
- Surgery is generally a last resort due to the loss of ability to perform self-care for a significant amount of time postoperatively.

Consults

- Physical medicine and rehabilitation
- Orthopedic surgery

Complications of treatment

- GI and renal complications from NSAIDs
- Lack of exercise if a power wheelchair is substituted for manual one.

Prognosis

- Poor, unless the underlying exacerbating activities are modified.

Helpful Hints

- Prescribe a balanced shoulder-strengthening program before shoulder pain begins.

Suggested Readings

Dyson-Hudson TA, Kirshblum SC. Shoulder pain in chronic spinal cord injury, Part I: Epidemiology, etiology and pathomechanics. *J Spinal Cord Med.* 2004;27(1):4–17.

Paralyzed Veterans of America Consortium for Spinal Cord Medicine. Preservation of upper limb function following spinal cord injury: A clinical practice guideline for healthcare professionals. *J Spinal Cord Med.* 2005;28(5):434–470.

Section I: Conditions

Neuropathic Pain: At and Below Level

Thomas N. Bryce MD ■ Igor Rakovchik DO

Description

Pain that arises as a direct consequence of a lesion or disease affecting the somatosensory system at the level of the spinal cord or nerve roots.

Etiology/Types

At Level

- Spinal cord (or central) pain
- Radicular (or nerve root) pain

Below Level

- Spinal cord (or central) pain

Epidemiology

- The prevalence of pain after SCI is between 65% and 80%, 20% to 30% of which is severe.
- 33% of pain after SCI at 2 weeks postinjury is neuropathic.
- 60% of pain after SCI at 6 months postinjury is neuropathic.

Pathogenesis

- By definition, at-level and below-level spinal cord pain arises from an initial injury to the spinal cord.
- Abnormal spontaneous and evoked electrical activity has been recorded in both the spinal cord and thalamus.
- Neuronal reorganization in the thalamus of persons with SCI and pain has been shown to occur.
- Increased sodium channel expression within pain-signaling neurons causes exaggerated nociceptive signaling.
- Transcortical dysrhythmia characterized by a shift in the dominant electroencephelographic spectral power peak is seen in persons with SCI and pain.
- Sprouting may explain the allodynia that is common in the dermatomes innervated by the damaged roots.

Risk Factors

- Unrelieved neural compression
- Depression

Clinical Features

At-level radicular pain

- At the neurologic level of injury (NLI) or within three dermatomes below this level: typically unilateral
- Characterized as stabbing, shooting, or electric shock-like (can be burning or aching)
- Temporally paroxysmal
- ± Hyperesthesia, hypoesthesia, allodynia, or analgesia

At-level spinal cord pain

- At the NLI or within three dermatomes below this level: typically bilateral
- Characterized as tightness, pressure, burning, cold
- Temporally continuous
- ± Allodynia or hyperalgesia

Below-level spinal cord pain

- Must occur in a region more than three dermatomes below the NLI, although the same pain can be localized within the three dermatomes below the NLI
- Characterized as burning, aching, numbness, pins and needles, cold, heaviness, or pressure
- Temporally continuous
- Allodynia or hyperalgesia can be present in those with some preserved sensation in the area of pain.

Natural History

- May develop immediately after injury, gradually over the course of weeks to months after injury, or years after injury

Diagnosis

Differential diagnosis

- Mechanical/musculoskeletal pain
- Visceral pain

History

- Unilateral or bilateral dermatomal distribution
- Burning, lancinating, or electric-like qualities
- Spinal cord pain usually is constant and not aggravated by movement or position change, although it can vary in intensity.

Exam

- Exam may be normal except for stigmata of SCI
- Allodynia to dynamic touch at area of pain
- Hyperalgesia to repetitive pinprick at area of pain

Testing

- MRI/CT may be helpful in ruling out syringomyelia, tumors, hardware loosening.

Pitfalls
- May be very difficult to differentiate from other pain syndromes
- Neuropathic pain can lead to nociceptive pain.

Red Flags
- New onset of pain after a delay may indicate syringomyelia or other cause of late neurologic decline.

Treatment

Medical
- Anticonvulsants (gabapentin, pregabalin, carbamazepine)
- Tricyclic antidepressants (amitryptyline)
- Selective serotonin and norepinephrine reuptake inhibitors
- Opioids (oral, transdermal, and intrathecal)
- Neurotoxins (intrathecal zoconotoxin)

Exercises
- Increase activity
- Desensitization techniques for evoked pain
- Biofeedback
- Hypnosis
- Cognitive behavioral therapy

Injection
- Transforaminal epidural steroid injections can be useful for radicular pain.

Surgical
- Decompression and spine stabilization if warranted
- Intrathecal pump implantation
- Dorsal root entry zone microcoagulation
- Spinal cord stimulators

Consults
- Physical medicine and rehabilitation
- Pain medicine
- Neuropsychology

Complications of treatment
- Medication side effects
- Loss of sensation with dorsal root entry zone procedure

Prognosis
- Poor without treatment
- Fair with treatment unless pain generator can be removed before secondary plastic neurologic changes occur

Helpful Hints
- Use a multimodal approach
- Treat early and aggressively

Suggested Readings
Bryce T, Ragnarsson, KT. Pain management in persons with spinal cord disorders. In: Lin V, ed. *Spinal Cord Medicine: Principles and Practice*. New York: Demos, 2003:441–460.

Widerström-Noga E, Biering-Sørensen F, Bryce T, et al. The International Spinal Cord Injury Pain Basic Data Set. *Spinal Cord*. 2008;46(12):818–823.

Section I: Conditions

Nontraumatic Spinal Cord Injury

Anousheh Behnegar MD ■ Kristjan T. Ragnarsson MD

Description

SCI that is not a direct result of a specific incurred mechanical trauma to the cord.

Etiology/Types

■ Cord compression
 – Stenosis
 – Tumor
 – Epidural abscess
 – Disk herniation/rupture
■ Vascular ischemia
 – Dissecting aortic aneurysm
 – Surgical procedures on the aorta
 – Decompression sickness
■ Vascular malformations causing compression and/or steal
■ Intraspinal hemorrhage
 – Vascular malformation
 – Coagulopathies
 – Tumor
 – Idiopathic
■ Infection
 – Viral
 – Bacterial
 – Fungal
 – Parasitic
■ Inflammation
 – Lupus
 – Sarcoid
■ Demyelinating diseases, eg, multiple sclerosis
■ Electric shock
■ Genetic
■ Vitamin B_{12} deficiency
■ Paraneoplastic

Epidemiology

■ Nontraumatic SCI accounts for one-third of acute SCI rehabilitation admissions.
■ Nontraumatic SCI is associated with older age (31% of persons younger than 40% and 87% of persons older than 40) and female gender, in contrast to traumatic SCI.
■ Spinal stenosis and tumors account for most nontraumatic SCI requiring acute inpatient rehabilitation.

Pathogenesis

■ Cord compression
■ Ischemia
■ Demyelination
■ Hemorrhage
■ Cystic necrosis

Risk Factors

■ Spinal stenosis
■ Neoplastic disease
■ Older age
■ Immunosuppression
■ Genetic predisposition

Clinical Features

■ Neurologic impairment associated with nontraumatic SCI is usually less severe than traumatic SCI.
■ Paraplegia is much more likely than tetraplegia.
■ Motor-incomplete SCI more likely than complete SCI
■ Slow onset of symptoms
■ Most often associated with history of spondylosis, rheumatoid arthritis, or neoplastic disease
■ Neoplastic cord compression involves the thoracic and lumbar regions more frequently than the cervical region.

Natural History

■ Lack of treatment can lead to increasing weakness and sensory loss.
■ Complications of an untreated neurogenic bladder and bowel can include UTIs, ureteral reflux, urolithiasis, renal failure, stool impaction, rectal bleeding, and hemorrhoids.
■ Pressure ulcers, orthostatic hypotension, spasticity, pain, respiratory insufficiency, pneumonia, thromboemboli, osteoporosis, sexual dysfunction, and depression can also occur.

Diagnosis

Differential diagnosis

■ Traumatic SCI
■ Various other neurologic conditions

History
- Progressive neurologic symptoms and signs such as weakness, sensory and motor deficits, bowel and bladder dysfunction
- Spinal stenosis
- Neoplastic disease
- Recent viral illness
- Recent travel to an underdeveloped area
- Pain when supine
- Intravenous drug use
- Recent injections
- Recent spinal surgery

Exam
- Complete physical and neurologic examination including an ASIA motor and sensory exam to determine neurologic level and degree of impairment
- Findings on exam that are associated with the underlying cause of the SCI such as the stigmata of a connective tissue disease

Testing
- X-rays and CT scans may show spondylosis and spinal stenosis if this is a cause.
- MRI can reveal cord abnormalities.
- Laboratory tests to include blood and CSF samples for cytology, chemical and microbiological testing, as well as blood tests for vitamin B_{12} levels, sedimentation rate, and rheumatoid factor.

Pitfalls
- Misdiagnosing the actual cause of cord damage
- Underestimating risk of comorbidities

Treatment

Medical
- Pharmacotherapy for underlying etiology, eg, infection, malignancy
- Prophylaxis and treatment of complications and comorbidities

Surgical
- Early decompression
- Shunting of CSF if applicable

Exercises
- Strengthening of innervated muscles
- ROM exercises for paralyzed limbs
- Training in ADLs, ambulation, wheelchair mobility, and transfers

Consults
- Physical medicine and rehabilitation
- Neurology
- Spine surgery
- Infectious disease
- Neurourology

Complications of treatment
- Organ toxicity from antibiotics or chemotherapy
- Failure of surgery
- Embolic vascular event after vascular imaging with contrast dye

Prognosis
- Neurologic and functional recovery depend on the level, extent and completeness of injury, and the success of the intervention and the nature of the disease.
- Functional recovery is generally comparable to traumatic SCI if there are no comorbidities and the length of rehabilitation stay is similar to that of traumatic SCI; otherwise, functional recovery is less favorable than traumatic SCI.

Suggested Readings

McKinley WO. Nontraumatic spinal cord injury: Etiology, incidence, and outcome. In: Kirshblum S, ed., *Spinal Cord Medicine*. Philadelphia: Lippincott Williams & Wilkins, 2002:471–479.

Woolsey RM, Martin D. Acute nontraumatic myelopathies and chronic nontraumatic myelopathies. In: Lin V, ed. *Spinal Cord Medicine: Principles and Practice*. New York: Demos, 2003:407–427.

Section I: Conditions

Obesity

Avniel Shetreat-Klein MD PhD

Description

Obesity carries increased risk factors for many comorbidities (diabetes, hyperlipidemia, hypertension) and affects the SCI population in greater proportion than the general public due to changes in activity and body composition.

Etiology/Types

- Obesity is defined as an excess of body fat.
- The World Health Organization (WHO) defines obesity as body mass index (BMI) >30 kg/m².
- Obesity can be further specified as moderate (30–35), severe (35 to 40), and very severe (>40 kg/m²).
- Other definitions include body fat of >22% for men or >35% for women.

Epidemiology

- Estimates of overweight or obesity range from 40% to 65% of the SCI population vs 30% of non-SCI population.

Pathogenesis

- Fundamentally, body fat (adipose) deposition is controlled by the balance between energy (calorie) intake and expenditure.
- Different nutrients have differing caloric density, but all can be converted to adipose tissue.
- Energy intake is controlled by appetite and satiety centers in the hypothalamus.
- Caloric expenditure can be divided into basal metabolic rate (BMR) and calories used for activity.
- BMR accounts for a 60% to 70% of total calorie expenditure.
- Of body tissues, skeletal muscle accounts for the greatest proportion of the BMR.
- Thus, in SCI, where there is atrophy of skeletal muscle due to loss of neurotrophic factors, BMR is decreased and energy balance is biased to excess intake.

Risk Factors

- Decreased energy expenditure, lower BMR, and skeletal muscle atrophy
- Hereditable component: over 600 gene products related to obesity have been identified.
- Environmental/psychological component plays a strong role.

- Obesity risk correlates with level and severity of injury.

Clinical Features

- Adipose tissue actively secretes cytokines including interleukin-6 and tumor necrosis factor α
- These cytokines are proinflammatory and lead to endothelial damage.
- Visceral body fat correlates with health risks more than subcutaneous fat.

Natural History

- Breakdown products from excess adipose tissue alter insulin and glucose pathways leading to glucose intolerance and insulin resistance.
- Accumulation of fatty acids in liver influences lipoprotein synthesis, leading to dyslipidemia.
- Hypertension can result in patients with obesity and SCI due to secretion of angiotensinogen from adipocytes, increased arterial stiffness, and mechanical compression of the kidneys.
- Obese patients with SCI are also more prone to musculoskeletal overuse injuries (particularly in the upper extremities).

Diagnosis

Differential diagnosis

- Medication effects (many psychotropic medications predispose to obesity)
- Hypothyroidism
- Hypothalamic injury
- Hypercortisolism
- Congenital

History

- While obesity often develops in SCI for the reasons noted, high prevalence of obesity in the general population implies that many cases of acquired SCI will be in patients already obese or with risk factors for obesity.

Exam

- Height, weight for BMI calculation
- Other mechanisms for calculating body fat percentage include skinfold testing, dual energy X-ray absorptiometry scan, or hydrostatic weighing. However, they are cumbersome and/or require specialized equipment

and training, and have not been validated specifically in patients with SCI.

Testing
- TSH
- Cortisol

Pitfalls
- Current studies indicate that BMI underestimates obesity in patients with SCI.
- Even when body weight does not change, lean body mass is reduced and body fat mass is increased proportionally.

Red Flags
- Risk of associated comorbidities increases exponentially with degree of obesity.

Treatment

Medical
- Mainstay of intake management is to keep total caloric intake between 100 and 200 calories below expenditure per day.
- Nutritionally dense foods that are low in cholesterol, saturated fats, and added salt and sugars can decrease "empty calories" and reduce food cravings.
- High glycemic index foods lead to hyperinsulinemia and glucose intolerance and should be avoided.

Exercises
- Increased caloric expenditure decreases caloric excess.

- Resistive exercise will also build skeletal muscle leading to enhanced BMR.

Consults
- Endocrinology
- Nutrition
- Psychology

Complications of treatment
- Rapid weight loss strategies preferentially cause loss of muscle stores, further lowering BMR, and do not reduce adiposity.

Prognosis
- The logical, empirical approach presented here is not yet supported by outcome studies.
- Extrapolating from obesity in non-SCI populations; long-term success in treating obesity requires very highly motivated patients and committed multidisciplinary treatment team.

Helpful Hints
- Prevention of obesity can be achieved with less effort than reversal of weight gain.

Suggested Readings
Chen Y, Henson S, Jackson AB, Richards JS. Obesity intervention in persons with spinal cord injury. *Spinal Cord.* 2006;44(2):82–91.

Gater DR, Jr. Obesity after spinal cord injury. *Phys Med Rehabil Clin N Am.* 2007;18(2):333–351.

Pediatric Spinal Cord Injury

Kristjan T. Ragnarsson MD

Description
Pediatric SCI occurs in persons under the age of 15 with SCI.

Etiology/Types
- Motor vehicle crashes
- Lap belt injuries
- Birth injury: 1/60,000 births
- Child abuse and violence
- Cranial vertebral junction injuries, often related to juvenile rheumatoid arthritis, Down syndrome, or skeletal dysplasia

Epidemiology
- SCI in young children is relatively rare, but incidence rises during adolescence.
- Less than 5% of all SCIs occur in children under the age of 15 (500/year in the United States).
- Boys and girls are equally affected among the youngest, but with rising age, boys are more often affected.

Pathogenesis
- Children have greater spinal mobility and less spinal stability than adults.
- SCI without radiological abnormalities (SCIWORA) is commonly seen in the youngest age group (60% in those under 10 years of age).
- SCIWORA is usually associated with neurologically complete lesions.
- Delayed onset of neurologic deficits (30 minutes to 4 days) occurs in 25% to 50% of children with SCI.

Risk Factors
- Insufficient restraint of children in cars
- Breach presentation at birth
- Developmental disorders
- Violent environment

Clinical Features
- Neurologic deficits associated with SCI
- Scoliosis
- Hip instability
- Reduced growth of paralyzed limbs
- Hypercalcemia during first 3 months after SCI

Natural History
- Neurologic recovery correlates in part to ASIA impairment score
- Scoliosis develops in 98% of children who sustain SCI prior to skeletal maturity, requiring surgery in 67%.
- Hip joint instability occurs in 60% to 100% of children injured before 8 years of age.
- Heterotopic ossification is rare (3%) compared to adults with SCI (20%).
- Complications can include UTIs, ureteral reflux, urolithiasis, urinary incontinence, pressure ulcers, stool incontinence or impaction, sexual dysfunction, spasticity, pain, autonomic dysreflexia, and respiratory impairment.

Diagnosis

Differential diagnosis
- Transverse myelitis
- Motor neuron disease
- Myopathy

History
- Sudden or delayed onset of neurological symptoms below a given neurologic level following trauma
- Urinary and bowel retention/incontinence
- No loss of consciousness or cognitive deficits in absence of head injury

Exam
- Perform general, physical, and neurologic examinations including the ASIA motor and sensory examination.
- Carefully assess spine, hips, and skin.

Testing
- X-rays may show no skeletal abnormality.
- MRI and CT abnormalities correlate with severity of the neurological deficit and skeletal injuries, respectively.

Pitfalls
- Normal imaging studies in children do not exclude SCI.
- Delayed onset of paralysis may occur after severe spinal injury in children.

Red Flags
- Decline in neurologic function

Treatment

Medical
- Acute SCI: consider high-dose methylprednisolone
- Clean intermittent catheterization is the standard bladder management for children.
- Deep venous thrombosis prophylaxis is the same as for adults.
- Spinal orthoses can prevent or correct scoliosis.
- Training in ADL, ambulation, and wheelchair mobility

Exercises
- Strengthening of innervated muscles
- ROM for paralyzed limbs
- Functional electrical stimulation ergometry for lower limb muscles

Surgical
- Early decompression and/or spinal stabilization
- Correction of scoliosis is indicated when curvature exceeds 40° in children over 10 years of age and >80° in those who are younger.
- Reconstructive surgery for hip joint subluxation or dislocation is controversial, but may include osteotomy or shelf arthroplasty.

Consults
- Physical medicine and rehabilitation
- Pediatrics
- Neurourology
- Spine surgery

Complications of treatment
- Failure of growth of instrumented areas
- Latex allergy from frequent and extensive contact with latex products

Prognosis
- Neurologic recovery depends on cord damage.
- Functional skills depend on neurologic level and completeness.
- Life expectancy is reduced.
- Psychosocial and vocational difficulties are common.

Helpful Hints
- As baseline blood pressures are typically lower in children, increases resulting from autonomic dysreflexia may be missed.
- Children may become febrile more readily with higher temperatures.
- Education, job training and employment, income, independent living, and good health are crucial for life satisfaction and need to be addressed early.

Suggested Readings
Howard H. Steel Conference on Pediatric Spinal Cord Injury. *Top Spinal Cord Inj Rehabil.* 2000:6(Suppl).
Vogel LC, Betz RR, Mulcahey MJ. Pediatric spinal cord disorders. In: Kirshblum S, Campanolo DI, DeLisa J, eds. *Spinal Cord Medicine.* Philadelphia: Lippincott Williams & Wilkins, 2002.

Pressure Ulcers

Donald Macron MD MA

Description
According to the National Pressure Ulcer Advisory Panel, a pressure ulcer "is localized injury to the skin and/or underlying tissue, usually over a bony prominence, as a result of pressure . . . shear and/or friction."

Etiology/Types
- Wounds develop from progressive tissue ischemia as well as from reperfusion injury.
- Severity depends primarily on degree and duration of pressure exerted and location.

Epidemiology
- Estimates among the SCI population range from one-quarter to as high as two-thirds of all individuals.
- Lifetime risk for persons with SCI is as high as 80%.
- Darker skin tone and higher level SCI lesions have been associated with increased incidence.

Pathogenesis
- Elevated tissue pressure prevents capillary perfusion, leading to cell death and necrosis.

Risk Factors
- Impaired sensation
- Impaired mobility
- Suboptimal nutrition
- Vascular disease, diabetes
- Altered mental status
- Incontinence and poor hygiene
- Exposure to shearing and friction forces
- Advanced age
- Hospitalization or institutionalization

Clinical Features
- Commonly involved regions include the ischium, sacrum, malleolus, scapula, greater trochanter, occiput, and heel.
- Staged using National Pressure Ulcer Advisory Panel system: stage I to stage IV depending on depth of tissue involvement, unstageable, and suspected deep tissue injury.

Natural History
- Stage I lesions: nonblanching erythema with intact skin

- Stage II wounds: superficial, "partial-thickness," often with bullae or shallow ulceration
- Stage III wounds: "full thickness skin loss," extension to the subcutaneous tissue
- Stage IV wounds: involvement of bone, muscle, joint, or other underlying structures; possible fistulae, sinus tracts, or undermining
- Unstageable wounds: due to coverage by slough or eschar
- Suspected deep tissue injury: localized area of purple or maroon skin due to damage to underlying soft tissue

Diagnosis

Differential diagnosis
- Infectious ulceration
- Venous stasis or arterial insufficiency
- Malignancy
- Traumatic wound or ulceration
- Thermal burn
- Diabetic ulceration
- Vascuilits, pyoderma gangrenosum, collagen vascular disease

History
- Inadequate positional changes in an immobilized or insensate person

Exam
- Regular whole-body assessments of skin integrity with emphasis on "at-risk" areas
- Note ulcer location, diameter, depth, stage, color, and drainage
- Photographs or clear-film tracings are useful for documentation.

Testing
- Bone scans, CT, and MRI are useful when warranted to assess involvement of underlying structures.
- Angiography, Doppler ultrasound, and other methods of assessing perfusion may be helpful.

Pitfalls
- Incorrect staging is common, especially if necrotic tissue or suspected deep tissue injury is present.

Treatment
- Prevention and minimization of risk factors are the cornerstone of treatment.

- Pressure mapping should be performed to identify areas at risk for breakdown.
- Appropriate wheelchair seating systems should be prescribed.
- Once formed, pressure relief and debridement is critical to healing wounds.
- Regular wound cleaning (eg, irrigating with dilute Dakin's solution or normal saline) reduces bacterial load.
- Consider surgical intervention for recurrent, nonhealing, infected, or poorly vascularized wounds.
- Wounds should be kept moist, and surrounding skin dry.
- Persons with or at risk for pressure ulcers require specialized support surfaces.
- Pressure relief maneuvers should occur at least every 20 minutes for 2 minutes in a wheelchair, and every 2 hours in bed.

Consults
- Physical medicine and rehabilitation
- Plastic surgery
- Infectious disease
- Nutrition

Complications of treatment
- Iatrogenic complications from debridement, flap surgery, and other manual interventions
- Adverse reactions from antibiotics, including neurotoxicity, renal toxicity, allergic and hypersensitivity reactions
- Fibroblast damage from corrosive solutions used in irrigation of wounds

Prognosis
- Depends on the severity of the wound(s), overall medical condition, and ability to prevent/eliminate causative agents.
- Early and aggressive intervention increases chances for healing.
- Education is essential to prevent recurrence.
- Pressure ulcers are themselves a risk factor for increased morbidity and mortality.

Helpful Hints
- Different tissues and regions have varied pressure sensitivities (muscle notably more susceptible than skin).
- ≥ 70 mm Hg pressure for ≥ 2 hours results in irreversible tissue damage.
- Up to 25% of SCI care costs relate to pressure ulcers.

Suggested Readings

Black J, Baharestani M, Cuddigan J, et al. National Pressure Ulcer Advisory Panel's updated pressure ulcer staging system. *Dermatol Nurs.* 2007;19(4):343–349.

Bluestein D, Javaheri A. Pressure ulcers: Prevention, evaluation and management. *Am Fam Phys.* 2008;78(10):1186–1194.

Consortium for Spinal Cord Medicine. Pressure ulcer prevention and treatment following spinal cord injury: A clinical practice guideline for health-care professionals. *J Spinal Cord Med.* 2001;24(Suppl 1):S40–S101.

Ho C, Bogie K. The prevention and treatment of pressure ulcers. *Phys Med Rehabil Clin N Am.* 2007;18(2):235–253.

Reddy M, Gill SS, Kalkar SR, et al. Treatment of pressure ulcers: A systematic review. *JAMA.* 2008;300(22):2647–2662.

Psychological Issues: Adjustment

Angela Riccobono PhD

Description
Adjustment or adaptation to SCI requires the indivdual to adapt to multiple life-altering losses, including movement; sensation; bowel, bladder and sexual function; job; self-image; and role in family. In short, adjustment to the loss of a previously known way of life.

Etiology/Types
- Positive adjustment
- Poor adjustment

Pathogenesis
- The adjustment process begins when individuals become aware that they have sustained a SCI.
- Poor adjustment often occurs when an individual is unable to pass through the initial stages of adjustment and remains "stuck" in a particular stage (eg, denial, anger, depressed mood).
  - Persons with poor adjustment are unable to acquire skills that promote independence, to set goals, and to realistically plan for future.
  - They are unable to achieve a satisfying quality of life and may have a lifestyle that is markedly different from premorbid lifestyle.
- In a good adjustment, the individual is able to set and achieve goals related to social, vocational, educational, and/or leisure pursuits.
  - Also able to reestablish satisfying social and intimate relationships and to "reinvent" an identity; one with meaning and purpose.

Risk Factors
Poor adjustment
- Substance/alcohol abuse
- Poor family and social support
- Limited/maladaptive coping strategies
- Psychiatric comorbidity
- Medical comorbidities
- Limited financial resources
- Lower education level
- TBI/cognitive problems
- Lack, or recent loss, of an intimate relationship
- Older age

Clinical Features
Poor adjustment
- Depression
- Anxiety
- Isolation
- Alcohol/substance abuse
- Poor self-care
- Inability to reintegrate into community

Natural History
- Individuals with a SCI will typically experience a period of grieving, which includes denial, anger, bargaining, sadness/depressed mood, and acceptance/accommodation.
  - Denial occurs when reality is too horrendous or disorganizing to absorb. In the rehabilitation setting, this often appears as a reluctance to carry out plans congruent with the disability, such as home modifications or avoiding therapy that suggests permanence, such as using adaptive equipment or splints. If not prolonged, denial can be positive, protecting the individual against depression and maintaining motivation.
  - In the anger phase, individuals shift from "not me" (denial) to "why me?," leading to verbal and physical outbursts. Anger can signify that the individuals acknowledge the injury and they are no longer in denial.
  - Bargaining is apparent in "if only" statements, such as "if only I had my hands."
  - Sadness/depressed mood is often a consequence of loss.
  - In acceptance/accommodation, the individuals begin integrating their injury into their life and setting realistic goals.

Diagnosis
Differential diagnosis
- It is important to distinguish the normal adjustment process from a pathologic adjustment.
- Individuals may grieve for up to a year or more as they grapple with adapting to a life altering injury.
- Individuals experiencing normal adjustment will focus emotions on issues directly related to the SCI

and loss of function, such as altered quality of life, loss of independence and control.

- These reactions should diminish over time as the individuals learn to integrate their disability into their life.
- An individual with poor adjustment will be self-critical, focused on feelings of hopelessness, helplessness, worthlessness, and withdrawal, and may meet the criteria for major depression.

History (poor adjustment)

- Inability to set/achieve goals regarding social, vocational, educational, or leisure activities
- Preoccupation with somatic complaints, including pain
- Inability to reestablish satisfying relationships, sexuality, and identity
- Social withdrawal
- Noncompliance with medications and self-care

Exam (poor adjustment)

- Disheveled appearance/neglect
- Depressed mood
- Flat affect
- Malnourished
- Multiple pressure sores
- Overly dependent on others
- Poor eye contact

Pitfalls

- Avoid overestimating psychological disturbance.

Red Flags

- Active alcohol/substance abuse
- Severe neglect
- Suicidal/homicidal ideation

Treatment

- Cognitive behavioral therapy aimed at reframing false assumptions and irrational beliefs, such as "I am less of a person because of my injury"
- Goal setting strategies
- Psychopharmacology
- Psychotherapy
- Support groups/peer mentoring

Prognosis

- Highly variable
- Mediated by premorbid individual traits and external factors
- Personality characteristics associated with positive adjustment include: optimism, humor, self-efficacy, and practical, solution-focused coping

Suggested Reading

Karp G, Klein SD. *From There to Here, Stories of Adjustment to Spinal Cord Injury*. Horsham, PA: No Limits Communications, 2004.

Section I: Conditions

Psychological Issues: Depression and Anxiety

Donald Macron MD MA

Description

Depression and anxiety are psychological disorders frequently resulting from, or exacerbated by, the experience of an SCI.

Etiology/Types

- Depression is at the core of a cluster of disorders, including major depressive disorder, dysthymia, bipolar disorder, schizoaffective disorder, and others.
- Anxiety disorders include generalized anxiety, obsessive-compulsive disorder, stress disorders [including posttraumatic stress disorder (PTSD)], panic disorders, and phobias.

Epidemiology

- Depressed mood may be universal post-SCI, but only some people develop full depressive disorders.
- Depression rates in the SCI population range from about 10% to 60%, depending on the criteria and definition.
- Anxiety is seen in 15% to 40% of people with SCI, particularly in acute and subacute settings.
- Anxiety and depression prevalence among people with SCI is significantly higher than the general population.

Pathogenesis

- Genetic, biological, social, and psychological factors predispose to anxiety and depression.
- The neurobiological genesis of depression and anxiety is unknown, but decreased levels of serotonin and norepinepherine have been posited.

Risk Factors

- History of depression or substance abuse prior to the SCI
- Chronic pain
- Female gender
- Family history
- Level of and completeness of spinal cord lesions do not correlate with depressive symptoms
- Depression, anxiety, stress, and PTSD appear linked in the SCI population; the presence of one increases the likelihood of others.

Clinical Features

- Depression features anhedonia, depressed mood, weight changes, sleep and psychomotor disturbances, concentration difficulties, intrusive thoughts, and fatigue.
- Fear, hypervigilance, autonomic overactivity, concentration difficulties, intrusive worrisome thoughts, and avoidant behavior are seen with anxiety disorders.

Natural History

- Anxiety and depression in the SCI population often manifests at around 30 weeks postinjury.
- Depressive and anxious symptoms within the first 12 weeks postinjury are associated with later recurrence.

Diagnosis

Differential diagnosis

- Anxiety and depressed mood are nonspecific symptoms: biological and alternative psychiatric diagnoses (eg, psychotic and delusional disorders, schizophrenia,) must be ruled-out.
- Adjustment disorder, bereavement, grief
- Endocrine, nutritional, and metabolic dysfunctions (eg, Addison's disease, thyroid disease, electrolyte imbalance, vitamin B_{12} deficiency, etc)
- Neurologic causes (eg, Alzheimer's dementia, Parkinson's disease, normal pressure hydrocephalus, etc)
- Substance-induced disorders and withdrawal syndromes
- Bipolar disorder

History

- Patients relate symptoms such as those listed in Clinical Features earlier.

Exam

- Depressed patients will often demonstrate flattened affect, tearfulness, or irritability and may have difficulty with attention, recall, and calculation.
- Anxiety can manifest in hypertension, diaphoresis, palpitations, headache, and stereotyped movements.

Testing
- Scales (such as the Beck Depression Inventory, State-Trait Anxiety Scale, and the Depression Anxiety and Distress Scale) are commonly used with persons with SCI; however, the reliability and sensitivity is variable.

Pitfalls
- The differential diagnosis for both depression and anxiety is long and complicated.
- Dual diagnoses—notably substance use/withdrawal, mood and dissociative disorders—must be carefully considered.

Treatment
- Pharmacologic and psychological treatment in tandem is the primary method for treating anxiety and depression, with the best success rate.
- Antidepressants and anxiolytics are frequently prescribed.
- Cognitive-behavioral therapy in particular has shown effectiveness in many depressed and anxious people.

Consults
- Psychology
- Neuropsychology
- Psychiatry

Complications of treatment
- Some antidepressants carry increased risk for suicidality with initiation of treatment.

- Serotonin reuptake inhibitors increase risk of serotonin syndrome.
- Antidepressants and particularly anxiolytics can be fatal if overdosed.
- Sedation and weight gain is associated with many agents.

Prognosis
- Early intervention improves prognosis.

Helpful Hints
- Persons with SCI in the acute setting should be screened for depression and anxiety, as early presentation correlates with worse prognosis.
- Reviewing pretraumatic mental health complaints as well as comorbidities is helpful in evaluation.

Suggested Readings
Martz E, Livneh H, Priebe M, et al. Predictors of psychosocial adaptation among people with spinal cord injury or disorder. *Arch Phys Med Rehabil.* 2005;86(6):1182–1192.

Osteråker AL, Levi R. Indicators of psychological distress in postacute spinal cord injured individuals. *Spinal Cord.* 2005;43(4):223–229.

Pollard C, Kennedy P. A longitudinal analysis of emotional impact, coping strategies and post-traumatic psychological growth following spinal cord injury: A 10-year review. *Br J Health Psychol.* 2007;12:347–362.

Section I: Conditions

Psychological Issues: Posttraumatic Stress Disorder

Donald Macron MD MA ■ Angela Riccobono PhD

Description

PTSD after SCI is a psychiatric anxiety-type disorder resulting from exposure to a severely traumatic stressor that involves actual or threatened death or serious injury or a threat to the physical integrity of self or others.

Etiology/Types

- An SCI may be the triggering stressor for developing PTSD, but can also be a coincidental event or compounding factor.
- PTSD is categorized as acute or chronic with symptoms lasting less than or greater than 3 months, respectively.
- Delayed-onset type PTSD can appear 6 months or longer after the inciting trauma.

Epidemiology

- Recent estimates put PTSD prevalence at 10% to 40% of the SCI population, compared with approximately 5% to 10% of the general U.S. population.
- Women have a higher incidence of PTSD than men, both in the general adult population and in the SCI population.
- The disorder affects all ages, and does not seem to have a racial predisposition.
- There is increased incidence among those with close relatives who have had PTSD, anxiety, or major depression.

Pathogenesis

- Several studies suggest that in PTSD, trauma is linked to changes in the amygdala, hippocampus, and speech and language centers.
- The stressor can be a personal experience—an event that involves or is witnessed by the patient—or learning about unexpected harm to a close associate or loved one.

Risk Factors

- History of prior trauma or abuse, particularly rape
- Shy or introverted personality
- Fire or motor vehicle accident involved with injury
- Paraplegia (increased risk compared to tetraplegia)

- Prior mental health conditions, particularly borderline and dependent personality disorders
- Severity and duration of the traumatic event correlate to risk

Clinical Features

- PTSD results in three broad symptom clusters: persistent re-experiencing, avoidant/numbness responses, increased arousal.
- People with PTSD re-experience their traumatic event through intrusive thoughts, nightmares, flashbacks, and physical reactions to triggers that symbolize the event.
- People exhibit avoidant/numbness responses by avoidance of activities, places, or people that remind the person of the trauma, diminished interest in activities, feelings of detachment or estrangement from others, and restricted range of feelings.
- People display hypervigilence and hyperarousal, such as sleeplessness, exaggerated startle response, anger outbursts, and difficulty concentrating.

Natural History

- Symptom resolution usually occurs over a 12- to 16-week period post-trauma, although relapses are common and symptoms may persist.
- Persistence of symptoms is related to severity of initial traumatic event.

Diagnosis

Differential diagnosis

- Adjustment disorder
- Other anxiety disorders
- Schizophrenia, particularly with intrusive thoughts
- Depressive disorders
- Substance-induced disorders
- Obsessive-compulsive disorder

History

- Exposure to traumatic event
- Development of symptoms lasting >4 weeks and associated with a decline in social, occupational, or other important areas of functioning

- Response must involve "intense fear, helplessness, or horror."
- Response in children must involve "disorganized or agitated behavior."

Exam
- Signs of increased autonomic arousal may be noted and monitored, but is generally not tested.

Testing
- Keane Scale, the Clinician-Administered PTSD Scale, and the Post-Traumatic Stress Diagnostic Scale

Pitfalls
- Dual diagnoses—particularly anxiety, substance abuse, sleep, and mood disorders—are common in this population and should be addressed.

Treatment
- Serotonin-norepinepherine reuptake inhibitors/ selective serotonin reuptake inhibitors, tricyclic antidepressants, and hypnotics are used for treatment.
- Cognitive-behavioral therapy has been shown to be effective for some.
- Psychodynamic psychotherapy is also used for treatment, although evidence is lacking for efficacy.

Consults
- Psychology
- Psychiatry

Complications of treatment
- Many medications used for PTSD have potential adverse side effects, including abuse.

Prognosis
- Early intervention improves prognosis.
- Relapsing and delayed-onset PTSD have a worse prognosis for eventual cure.

Helpful Hints
- Clinicians should be alert in the acute setting to recognize PTSD early.
- Pharmacologic and psychological treatment in tandem is considered the most effective treatment.

Suggested Readings

U.S. Department of Veterans Affairs. National Center for Posttraumatic Stress Disorder. Available at www.ncptsd.org/

Kennedy P, Duff J. Post traumatic stress disorder and spinal cord injuries. *Spinal Cord.* 2001;39:1–10.

Nielsen MS. Post-traumatic stress disorder and emotional distress in persons with spinal cord lesion. *Spinal Cord.* 2003;41:296–302.

Section I: Conditions

Pulmonary Issues: Atelectasis, Pneumonia, and Pleural Effusions

Thomas N. Bryce MD

Description

Atelectasis refers to the collapse of alveoli. Pneumonia commonly occurs in areas of atelectasis while pleural effusions often develop in close proximity.

Etiology/Types

- Decreased diaphragmatic muscle strength leads to incomplete lung expansion.
- Obstruction of small airways by excess secretions prohibits full lung expansion.

Epidemiology

- Pulmonary complications, including atelectasis, pneumonia, and pleural complications, are the leading causes of death for persons with SCI.
- Pulmonary complications account for approximately 40% of all deaths during the first year after SCI, and 20% of the deaths beyond the first year.
- 60% of persons with a C3 or C4 SCI on a ventilator upon transfer to a tertiary care facility have atelectasis.

Pathogenesis

- The development of atelectasis is related to weakness of respiratory muscles especially the diaphragm not allowing adequate expansion of affected alveoli.
- Decreased thoracic wall compliance is caused by chronic inexpansion or spasticity.
- Airway hyper-reactivity is thought to be caused by unopposed cholinergic tone.
- Pleural effusions occur near areas of atelectatic lung, which pull the parietal pleura away from the visceral pleura leaving an empty space that fills with fluid.

Risk Factors

- Mechanical ventilation
- Diaphragmatic/phrenic pacing
- Cervical and thoracic level SCI with weakness of the intercostals and abdominal muscles

Clinical Features

- The most common location for atelectasis is the left lower lobe.

Natural History

- Pneumonia will often develop in areas of untreated atelectatic lung.
- Pleural effusions will often occur adjacent to areas of atelectatic lung.
- Pleural effusions can become infected resulting in empyema.
- Pneumonia and empyema can lead to respiratory failure, sepsis, and death.

Diagnosis

Differential diagnosis

- Tracheobronchitis
- Upper respiratory infection
- Pulmonary embolus
- CHF

History

- Shortness of breath
- Increasing anxiety related to breathing
- Increased volume of secretions
- Increased frequency of suctioning
- Increased tenacity of secretions

Exam

- Increasing pulse rate
- Elevated temperature
- Increasing respiratory rate
- Rhales, rhonchi, and wheezing on auscultation

Testing

- Check vital capacity and negative inspiratory force as proxies for respiratory muscle strength.
- Peak expiratory flow rate
- Pulse oximetry
- Chest radiograph
- CT angiogram or ventilation perfusion scan to evaluate for pulmonary embolus

Pitfalls

- Not treating atelectasis aggressively can lead to pneumonia and pleural effusions.
- Overuse of broad spectrum antibiotics can lead to drug resistance.

Red Flags

- Respiratory failure
- Sepsis

Treatment

Medical

- An abdominal binder allows a more efficient diaphragmatic resting position.
- Bronchodilators reduce airway hyper-reactivity and constriction.
- Mucolytics and hydration loosen tenacious secretions.
- Postural drainage and chest percussion to mobilize secretions
- Manually assistive cough and mechanical insufflation-exsufflation to clear secretions
- Bronchoscopy to clear secretions for persistant atelectasis or lung collapse
- Intermittent positive-pressure breathing (IPPB), bilevel positive airway pressure (BiPAP), or continuous positive airway pressure (CPAP) prevent atelectasis.
- Increased ventilated tidal volumes to a target of >20 cc/kg ideal body weight prevent atelectasis.

Exercises

- Deep breathing exercises
- Incentive spirometry
- Resistive inspiration

Modalities

- Mechanical vibrator for secretion mobilization
- Vibrating vest for secretion mobilization

Surgical

- Tracheostomy placement to facilitate suctioning

Consults

- Pulmonary medicine

Complications of treatment

- Antibiotic resistance from indiscriminant use of antibiotics
- Pneumothorax from high airway pressures occurring from use of high tidal volumes
- Tachycardia from use of beta-adrenergic drugs
- Hemoptysis and airway trauma from overly aggressive suctioning

Prognosis

- Atelectasis and atelectasis-related pneumonia and pleural effusions are typically preventable and treatable with appropriate care.

Helpful Hints

- Treat atelectasis aggressively to prevent atelectasis-related pneumonia and pleural effusions

Suggested Readings

Bryce TN, Ragnarsson KT, Stein AS. Spinal cord injury. In: Braddom RL, ed. *Physical Medicine and Rehabilitation*. 3rd ed. Philadelphia: Saunders Elsevier, 2007:1285–1349.

Cosortium for Spinal Cord Medicine. Respiratory management following spinal cord injury: a clinical practice guideline for health-care professionals. *J Spinal Cord Med*. 2005;28(3):259–293.

Section I: Conditions

Sexuality and Reproductive Issues: Erectile Dysfunction

Naomi Betesh DO

Description

Erectile dysfunction (ED) is the inability to achieve or sustain an erection for satisfactory sexual intercourse. In people with SCI, sexual functioning is dependent on level and extent of injury.

Etiology/Types

- Reflexogenic
- Psychogenic
- Mixed erection

Epidemiology

- Some type of ED occurs in 75% of individuals with SCI.
- Erection more likely to be obtained in persons with incomplete SCI.
- Approximately 10% of ED in persons with SCI is psychogenic.

Pathogenesis

- Reflex erection occurs when a sensory stimulus in the genitals triggers a reflex arc, which travels through parasympathetics at S2-S4.
- Psychogenic erection can also be triggered via stimuli perceived in the brain via sympathetic center at T10-L2 spinal cord segments.
- Ability to have a reflexogenic or psychogenic erection after SCI depends on whether these pathways are intact.

Risk Factors

- Complete injury
- Co-morbid conditions including vascular causes, hormonal imbalances, other neurologic disorders
- Trauma or surgery to pelvic region
- Medications that effect erection

Clinical Features

- No specific clinical features; diagnosis is made solely by history of an inability to attain or sustain an erection sufficient for sexual intercourse.

Natural History

- Persons with UMN lesions are generally able to achieve reflexogenic erections.
- Persons with LMN lesions are unable to achieve reflex erections but may be able to achieve psychogenic erections.
- In either case, the erections are of poor quality and not sustainable.

Diagnosis

Differential diagnosis

- Vascular causes
- Iatrogenic secondary to prostate, bladder, or sphincter surgery
- Medication related
- Hormonal imbalance
- Other neurologic causes
- Psychological causes

History

- Neurologic classification of SCI
- Presence of chronic disease that may play a role
- Medication that may contribute
- History of substance abuse or mood disorder
- History of abdominal/pelvic trauma or surgery
- Sexual history to include ability to have and sustain erections, under what circumstances, presence of ED prior to injury
- Social history including stressors

Exam

- Genital exam to help rule out endocrine or genital disorder contributing to ED
- Sensory exam
- Bulbocavernosis reflex and anal cutaneous reflex

Testing

If etiology unclear, can consider the following tests dependent on history and physical exam.

- Nocturnal penile tumescence monitoring
- Doppler ultrasound to assess vascular flow to penis
- Fasting blood glucose
- Lipid profile
- Testosterone levels—free or total—if decreased then check luteinizing hormone and prolactin
- Thyroid tests

Pitfalls

- In spinal cord injured individuals with lesions above T6 penile sexual stimulation can lead to autonomic dysreflexia.

Red Flags

- Erection lasting >3 hours
- Infection

Treatment

Medical

- Oral PDE5 inhibitors
- Sexual counseling
- Intraurethral alprostadil suppositories

Exercises

- General conditioning
- Genital stimulation in those with some erectile function

Modalities

- Vacuum devices

Injection

- Intercavernous injection of vasoactive drugs

Surgical

- Penile prosthesis
- Sacral root stimulation

Consults

- Physical medicine and rehabilitation
- Urology

Complications of treatment

- Penile fibrosis
- Priapism with intracavernous injection therapy

- Autonomic dysreflexia
- Syncope with alprostadil
- Pain after injection
- Penile skin necrosis
- Infection or erosion of the prosthesis through the skin or urethra

Prognosis

- Majority of patients will be able to sustain an erection sufficient for intercourse with oral PDE5 inhibitors regardless of cause of ED. Efficacy of other therapies varies.

Helpful Hints

- Worsening of ED in patient with known ED is usually secondary to arterial or veno-occlusive disease.
- Vacuum devices and constriction rings can only be used for half an hour at a time to avoid penile ischemia
- Include patient's partner in discussion of choice of treatment.
- Do not prescribe vacuum devices or constriction rings for patients on anticoagulation.

Suggested Readings

Biering-Sorenson F, Sonksen J. Sexual function in spinal cord lesioned men. *Spinal Cord.* 2001;39(9):455–470.

Moemen MN, Fahmy I, AbdelAal M, et al. Erectile dysfunction in spinal cord injured men: different treatment options. *Int J Impot Res.* 2008;20(2):181–187.

Monga M, Bernie J, Rajasekaran M, et al. Male infertility and erectile dysfunction in spinal cord injury: review. *Arch Phys Med Rehabil.* 1999;80:1331–1339.

Ramos AS, Samso JV. Specific aspects of erectile dysfunction in spinal cord injury. *Int J Impot Res.* 2004;16:S42–S45.

Sexuality and Reproductive Issues: Pregnancy

Naomi Betesh DO

Description
Pregnancy after SCI presents a unique challenge due to the chronic medical conditions associated with SCI. All pregnancies in women with SCI should be considered high risk.

Etiology/Types
- Chronic SCI patients who conceive
- Acute SCI sustained during pregnancy

Epidemiology
- 1,000 new SCIs per year in females aged 16 to 30
- Few cases of SCI during pregnancy reported

Clinical Features
- Normal clinical features of pregnancy
- Asymptomatic bacteriuria occurs in most women with SCI during pregnancy.
- Urinary stasis due to changes in the normal anatomy of the urinary system increases the risk of UTIs, including pyelonephritis.
- Weight gain and edema, leading to improperly fitting equipment and inability to check skin properly may contribute to an increased risk for pressure ulcers.
- Women with high thoracic or cervical lesions may have impaired pulmonary function, which may be further impaired by decreased chest cavity space due to the increasing size of the fetus and supine lying.
- Women with spinal cord lesions at T6 or above are at risk for autonomic dysreflexia secondary to loss of hypothalamic control of sympathetic spinal reflexes.
- Theoretical risk of deep vein thrombosis and pulmonary edema due to pregnancy and SCI although not many cases have been reported.

Natural History
- Although there is limited data, pregnant women with SCI have been able to deliver healthy full-term babies.

Diagnosis

History
- Level and extent of injury
- Ability to care for self, including transfers, skin care, self-catheterize
- Bladder and bowel routine
- Expected due date, weeks gestation

Exam
- Routine skin exams with attention to proper fit of medical equipment
- Serial assessments of vital capacity may be indicated.
- Routine obstetric care
- Weekly cervical exams starting at 28 weeks and hospital admission once cervical dilation or effacement is noted in women with impaired uterine sensation.
- Topical anesthetics should be used prior to urethral, bladder, rectal, vaginal/cervical manipulation.

Testing
- Baseline pulmonary and renal function assessment may be indicated.
- All routine obstetrics testing
- Frequent urine surveillance cultures
- Monitor hemoglobin, hematocrit, iron studies

Pitfalls
- Hypotension, which is common in spinal cord injured individuals, may be aggravated by a hormonally mediated decrease in systemic vascular resistance due to pregnancy.
- With increasing weight gain of pregnancy, self-transfers become more difficult. Muscle atrophy and osteoporosis secondary to SCI can contribute to pathologic fractures.

Red Flags
- Autonomic dysreflexia uncontrolled by medical and pharmacologic intervention
- Presence of new unilateral lower extremity edema

Treatment

Medical
- Antibiotics for UTI as needed
- Avoid indwelling catheters if possible

- Minimize bladder residual volumes
- Iron supplementation for anemia
- Prescription of temporary or loaner power wheelchair
- Advise caregiver to assist with transfers

Exercises
- General ROM
- Strengthening exercises to upper extremities

Surgical
- Management of spine fractures during pregnancy should be determined on a case by case basis.

Consults
- Preconception evaluation
- Obstetrician specializing in high-risk pregnancy
- Anesthesia for ante partum evaluation prior to labor
- Occupational therapy for wheelchair and cushion evaluation
- Genetics if patient has congenital SCI

Complications of treatment
- Fetal abnormalities
- Spontaneous abortion or intrauterine death
- Death

Prognosis
- Patients with acute SCI during pregnancy may be at risk for spontaneous abortion, fetal malformation, abruption placentae, or direct fetal injury, depending on mechanism of trauma and resultant injuries.
- Patients with chronic acquired SCIs do not seem to be at greater risk for congenital malformations or intrauterine death.

Helpful Hints
- Treat women with acute SCI during pregnancy with at least 8 weeks of deep vein thrombosis prophylaxis.
- Refer women with congenital SCI to genetic counseling prior to pregnancy and start on folic acid.
- Advise pregnant women to change position slowly, because there is an increased risk for orthostatic hypotension.

Suggested Readings

ACOG Committee Opinion. Obstetric management of patients with spinal cord injuries. *Int J Gynecol Obstet.* 2002;79:189–191.

Kang AH, Traumatic Spinal cord injury. *Clin Obstet Gynecol.* 2005;48(1):67–72.

Pereira L. Obstetric management of the patient with spinal cord injury. *Obstet Gynecol Surv.* 2003;58(10):678–686.

Section I: Conditions

Sleep Apnea

Stephen Burns MD

Description
Sleep apnea is defined as an abnormal frequency of periods during sleep with cessation or reduction in airflow, typically defined as ≥10 seconds duration.

Etiology/Types
- Obstructive sleep apnea: if respiratory effort continues during apnea events. This is usually caused by upper airway collapse at level of retropalatal pharynx during inspiration.
- Central sleep apnea: if respiratory effort is absent/reduced during apnea events. This may occur if brain stem is affected (eg, syringobulbia) or possibly due to impaired afferent input from chest.
- Mixed: single apnea events may be mixed (central initially, changing to obstructive later in the episode) or combination of obstructive and central sleep apnea episodes.

Epidemiology
- Acute/subacute tetraplegia: 60% to 83% prevalence
- Chronic tetraplegia: 50% prevalence
- Paraplegia: poorly characterized
- Predominantly central sleep apnea pattern seen in 25%

Pathogenesis
- Apnea causes individual to wake from deeper to shallower stage of sleep.
- Sleep disruption leads to excessive daytime fatigue, cognitive impairment, risk for motor vehicle crashes.
- Stroke, cardiac disorders, systemic hypertension, and pulmonary hypertension are associated with sleep apnea through multiple mechanisms.

Risk Factors
- In general population, obesity is the most common risk factor for obstructive sleep apnea.
- Retrognathia and supine sleep position also associated.
- With SCI, additional risk factors include degree of neurological impairment affecting respiratory muscles and use of baclofen (mixed findings).

Clinical Features
- Excessive daytime sleepiness
- Observed apneas

Natural History
- Untreated sleep apnea persists unless risk factors are modified.

Diagnosis
Differential diagnosis
- Sleepiness has numerous causes in this population including sedating medications, sleep disruption from nursing care, and depression.

History
- Excessive daytime sleepiness
- Awakening with gasping or difficulty breathing
- Apneas or loud snoring reported by bed partners or hospital staff

Exam
- Exam findings are not sufficient to confirm diagnosis
- Elevated body mass index or large neck

Testing
- Polysomnography: includes airflow, respiratory effort, oxygen saturation, body position, and electroencephalography (EEG) to determine sleep stage. This may be performed in a sleep lab or with home monitoring.
- Limited polysomnography (without EEG) is less accurate but may available for use on hospital wards.

Pitfalls
- Conventional pulse oximeters may not detect short duration desaturation, due to averaging of readings, nor will it detect events that disrupt sleep without causing desaturation.
- Obstructive sleep apnea can indicate severe respiratory muscle weakness, requiring assessment of arterial carbon dioxide. These people should be managed with noninvasive ventilation.

Treatment
Medical
- CPAP or BiPAP delivered through nasal or oronasal mask are the treatment of choice for obstructive sleep apnea.
- Central sleep apnea often requires BiPAP with a back-up set rate

- Oral appliance (dual "retainer plates" that pull jaw anteriorly and open the airway)
- Weight loss (for obese persons) and avoidance of supine sleeping position can reduce apneas.

Surgical

- Uvulopalatopharyngoplasty: 50% success reported in general population. Other surgeries are sometimes indicated.

Consults

- Sleep medicine specialist (typically pulmonologist or neurologist)
- Otolaryngology if surgery is considered

Complications of treatment

- Discomfort from mask
- Surgical complications

Prognosis

- Most people will tolerate CPAP or BiPAP and have a significant reduction in apnea frequency and duration.

- Sleepiness and other cognitive symptoms usually improve with successful treatment.

Helpful Hints

- People with weak respiratory muscles may have difficulty breathing against a high CPAP pressure. BiPAP is preferred for these people, with "wide span" between inspiratory and expiratory pressures.
- To optimize CPAP/BiPAP acceptance, an occupational therapist should assess and modify equipment for those with impaired upper limb strength.

Suggested Readings

Berlowitz DJ, Brown DJ, Campbell DA, Pierce RJ. A longitudinal evaluation of sleep and breathing in the first year after cervical spinal cord injury. *Arch Phys Med Rehabil.* 2005;86(6):1193–1199.

Burns SP, Yavari Rad M, Bryant S, Kapur V. Long-term treatment of sleep apnea in persons with spinal cord injury. *Am J Phys Med Rehabil.* 2005;84(8):20–26.

Stockhammer E, Tobon A, Michel F, et al. Characteristics of sleep apnea syndrome in tetraplegic patients. *Spinal Cord.* 2002;40(6):286–294.

Section I: Conditions

Spasticity

Donald Macron MD MA

Description
Spasticity is characterized by a velocity-dependent increase in muscle tone.

Etiology/Types
- Spasticity results from an UMN injury.
- The Modified Ashworth scale can be used to grade the degree of spasticity:
  - 0: No spasticity
  - 1: Slight increase in resistance to ROM not sustained
  - 1+: Increased resistance sustained for less than half the ROM
  - 2: Increased tone throughout ROM, but limb easily moved
  - 3: Passive movement difficult
  - 4: Affected parts rigid to ROM

Epidemiology
- Frequent in the SCI population, with estimates as high as 60% to 80%
- There is a positive correlation between spasticity and completeness of injury

Pathogenesis
- After SCI, spasticity originates from decreased cortical inhibitory input due to damage to the UMN.
- Decreased afferent input to the central nervous system (CNS) is likely to play a role as well.

Risk Factors
- CNS insult (UMN damage) is the primary risk factor for spasticity.
- Conditions such as infection, venous thrombosis, trauma, syringomyelia, and stress can all increase spasticity.

Clinical Features
- Velocity-dependent increased muscle tone, in response to passive stretch
- Clonus
- Hyper-reflexia
- Hyperactive responses to external or internal stimuli

Natural History
- *Spinal shock* can last from several days to 6 weeks. It is characterized by muscle hypotonia and hyporeflexia.
- A *transitional phase* follows, with a progressive increase in tone, reflexive response, and spasm frequency.
- The *spastic state* (usually by 2 to 6 months postinjury) often shows plateauing of spasticity, though it may wax and wane in response to various conditions.

Diagnosis
Differential diagnosis
- Contracture
- Parkinsonism
- Stroke
- Medication withdrawal

History
- History of UMN injury
- The Penn Spasm Frequency Score is commonly used to quantify phasic spasticity

Exam
- Affected limbs will show a velocity-related "catch" and resistance to passive ROM
- "Soft" end-feel to ROM
- The Ashworth or Modified Ashworth scales are frequently used to describe tonic spasticity

Pitfalls
- Individual presentation is variable and can change with a number of factors, including time of day, inciting stimuli, and position
- Therefore sequential exams and self-descriptions are essential to evaluation.

Red Flags
- A new change in a previously stable spasticity workup may indicate a new medical condition such as syrinx, infection, or deep vein thrombosis.

Treatment
Medical
- Baclofen, a gamma-aminobutyric acid (GABA) analog, can be administered orally, or intrathecally

via implanted pump (potentially reducing dose-limiting side effects).

- Alpha-2 adrenergic agonists (eg, tizanidine, clonidine) inhibit neurotransmission.
- Benzodiazepines, as GABA facilitators, act to increase presynaptic inhibition of motor neurons.

Exercises
- Stretching and ROM exercises decrease spasticity and can prevent contractures.
- Positioning (eg, frog leg) can reduce spasticity or break a spasm.

Injections
- Up to 6 months of relief can be achieved by chemical neurolysis via alcohol, phenol, or botulinum toxin injection.

Consults
- Physical medicine and rehabilitation
- Neurosurgery for intrathecal baclofen pump placement

Complications of treatment
- Medications used for spasticity have potential dependence, sedation, or hypotensive side effects.
- Resistance to neurotoxins can develop with repeated administrations.

- Intrathecal pumps require surgical implantation and ongoing maintenance, both of which have risks.

Prognosis
- If left untreated, can lead to contracture, progressive deformity, and loss of function.

Helpful Hints
- Several factors, such as bowel/bladder dysfunction, autonomic dysreflexia, infection, pressure ulcers, renal calculi, DVT, temperature extremes, malpositioning, can incite or exacerbate spasticity in an SCI patient.
- Spasticity is not always problematic; it can have no impact or even be useful (as when used to assist patient mobility and positioning).
- Self report is key to assessing spasticity; the waxing and waning nature of the symptoms limit the usefulness of clinician observation and exam.

Suggested Readings
Hsieh JT, Wolfe DL, Miller WC, et al. Spasticity outcome measures in spinal cord injury: Psychometric properties and clinical utility. *Spinal Cord.* 2008;46(2):86–95.

Maynard FM, Waring WP, Karunas RS. Epidemiology of spasticity following traumatic spinal cord injury. *Arch Phys Med Rehabil.* 1990;71(8):566–569.

Sheean G. The pathophysiology of spasticity. *Eur J Neurol.* 2002;9(S1):3–9.

Section I: Conditions

Spinal Fractures

Justin T. Hata MD

Description
Spinal fractures can be stable or unstable, depending on what elements of the spine are disrupted.

Etiology/Types
- A burst fracture is a comminuted vertebral body fracture with spread of fragments in all directions.
- A compression fracture is a comminuted fracture of the anterior portion of the vertebral body only.
- A burst fracture of C1, or Jefferson fracture, is the most common fracture at C1.
- Odontoid fracture is most common at the junction of odontoid process and the body of C1.
- Traumatic spondylolisthesis of C2, or Hangman's fracture, typically is unstable.
- Thoracolumbar transverse fracture, or Chance fracture, is a horizontal fracture through the spinous process and the vertebral body.
- Isolated spinous process, lamina, and transverse process fractures

Epidemiology
- Motor vehicle accidents (45%), falls (20%), sports (15%), violent acts (15%)
- Incidence of C1–C2 fractures progressively rises with age
- Fifty percent of all vertebral body fractures occur between T11 and L2
- Male to female ratio is 4:1 for spine trauma in population <65 years
- Falls most common mechanism in elderly

Pathogenesis
- Vertebral body compression and burst fractures are due to axial compression.
- A severe flexion force usually results in a stable anterior wedge compression fracture.
- A Jefferson fracture is due to axial loading with flexion or extension.
- An odontoid fracture is due to flexion or extension forces.
- Flexion-rotation can produce a highly unstable injury, with ruptured posterior ligaments.
- Shear can result in spondylolisthesis.

- A Chance fracture is a flexion-distraction lesion, usually at L1–L3, which is acutely unstable, but has excellent healing potential.
- An extension injury may result in facet, lamina, or spinous process fractures.

Risk Factors
- Trauma
- High-energy impact activities
- Osteoporosis, especially with prior fracture
- Malignancy within bone
- Spondylopathies
- Age

Clinical Features
- Neck or back pain
- Neurologic deficits
- Paresthesias

Natural History
- Complete cord injuries and neurologically intact patients likely to remain neurologically unchanged with appropriate care.
- Nonunion is likely with nonoperative treatment of transverse type 2 and posterior displaced odontoid fractures.

Diagnosis
Differential diagnosis
- Dislocation or subluxation
- Whiplash injury
- Paraspinal muscle spasm
- Osteomyelitis

History
- Trauma: motor vehicle accident, fall, diving, sports injury
- Neck or back pain
- Neurologic deficit

Exam
- Anatomic deformity on inspection
- Localized tenderness
- Abdominal contusion caused by a lap belt may indicate a flexion-distraction injury
- Neurologic deficit

Testing
- CT is more sensitive than X-ray.
- Neck trauma X-rays should include anteroposterior (AP), odontoid, and lateral views of the C-T junction.
- MRI indicated for neurologic injury and when surgery is being considered.

Pitfalls
- 25% of burst fractures may be misdiagnosed as stable wedge fractures by plain radiographs.
- From 50% to 60% of spine-injured patients have associated nonorthopedic injury.

Red Flags
- Unstable fracture
- Posterior ligamentous injury
- Neurologic deficit

Treatment

Medical
- Stable cervical fractures usually treated with a halo or hard collar
- Unstable Jefferson fractures treated with traction then halo
- Spinal orthoses

Exercises
- Extension program for osteoporosis or kyphotic deformities

Modalities
- Bone stimulator

Injections
- Vertebroplasty or kyphoplasty for symptomatic vertebral compression fractures

Surgical
- A C2 transverse type 2 odontoid and severe Hangman's fractures require surgery.
- Subaxial (C3–C7) vertebral body and facet fractures may require surgery based on stability.
- Surgery usually required for posterior ligamentous injuries, multiple compression fractures, and unstable fractures.

Consults
- Spine surgery

Complications of treatment
- Nonunion
- Pain
- Infection
- Worsening neurological deficit
- Hardware loosening

Prognosis
- C-spine fractures in elderly are often complicated by comorbidities and poor tolerance for immobilization.

Helpful Hints
- Burst fractures unstable: if neurologic deficit, >50% loss of vertebral body height, or >20° angulation with >30% canal compromise at T–L junction.
- C1 fractures rarely associated with neurologic deficit.

Suggested Readings
Bono CM, Vives MF, Kauffman CP. Cervical injuries: Indications and options for surgery. In: Lin VW, ed. *Spinal Cord Medicine: Principles and Practices*. New York: Demos, 2003:131–141.

Savas PE, Vaccaro AR. Surgical management for thoracolumbar spinal injuries. In: Lin VW, ed. *Spinal Cord Medicine: Principles and Practices*. New York: Demos, 2003:141–151.

Section I: Conditions

Spinal Instability

Kristjan T. Ragnarsson MD

Description

Spinal instability is the inability to limit excessive or abnormal spinal displacement, which can lead to neurologic deficit, deformity, and pain.

Etiology/Types

- Trauma resulting in two or three column fracture or extensive ligamental rupture
- Disease causing two or three column destruction or extensive ligamental rupture

Epidemiology

- Major trauma or disease affecting the cervical or lumbar spine, as well as the thoracolumbar junction of the spine, are often associated with spinal instability.
- The thoracic spine is the most stable segment of the vertebral column and least likely to be unstable due to its support from the rib cage, anatomical overlapping of the posterior elements, and strong spinal ligaments.

Pathogenesis

- Disruption of at least two of the three columns of the spine as described by Denis
- The anterior column: anterior vertebral body, anterior longitudinal ligament, and anterior half of the annulus fibrosus
- Middle column: posterior vertebral body, posterior longitudinal ligament, and posterior half of the annulus fibrosus
- Posterior column: posterior bone/ligament complex, including lamina, pedicles, supraspinous, intraspinous, and flavum ligaments

Risk Factors

- Two or three column spinal injury or ligamental disruption
- Trauma or disease affecting the cervical, lumbar, or thoracolumbar segments of the spine

Clinical Features

- Neck or back pain with motion
- Neurologic symptoms and/or signs with spinal motion, eg, motor loss, sensory deficits, bowel and bladder dyscontrol

Natural History

- Ligamental ruptures do not heal, and associated spinal instability will continue without surgical fusion.
- Fractures usually heal in time with proper spinal immobilization.

Diagnosis

Differential diagnosis

- Nontraumatic causes for SCI
- Variety of acquired neurologic conditions

History

- Spinal trauma
- Neck or back pain, especially with movement
- Neurologic impairment after trauma

Exam

- Localized tenderness over the spine
- Local paraspinal muscle spasm
- Pain with movement (suspected unstable areas should not be moved when there is a risk of neurologic compromise)
- Neurologic deficits

Testing

- Imaging studies: X-rays, CT scan, MRI
- Imaging evidence of two or three column injury
- Imaging studies that show translation of >25% of the width of the vertebra indicate three column disruption
- Flexion-extension imaging studies that show >3.5 mm sagittal displacement of one vertebra in relation to the adjacent vertebra or >11° angular tilt on sagittal flexion

Pitfalls

- Pain and muscle spasm can inhibit displacement and translation on dynamic imaging.

Red Flags

- Neurologic symptoms and signs on flexion, extension, or other spinal movement
- Deteriorating neurologic condition

Treatment

Medical

- Spinal immobilization is initially accomplished by placing the patient on a spinal board in supine position supported by appropriate external orthoses.

- Log roll side to side for skin inspection and comfort.
- Spinal traction may be applied to reduce fracture dislocation with locked facets or for a short-term spinal immobilization.
- For cervical spine immobilization: apply head-cervical-thoracic-orthoses (HCTO), eg, Halo vest or Minerva jacket, or when indicated, rigid head-cervical-orthoses (HCO), eg, Miami J, Philadelphia, or Aspen collars.
- For thoracolumbar fractures: apply thoracolumbosacral orthosis (TLSO).

Surgical

- Stabilization is usually preceded by decompression of neural structures
- Anterior or posterior approach
- Autologous bone grafts and/or implanted hardware for fixation during healing

Consults

- Spinal surgery

Complications of treatment

- Failure of surgical fixation
- Skin breakdown under orthoses

Prognosis

- Most spinal fractures heal with external stabilization, resulting in a stable spine.
- Severe ligamental disruptions do not heal, and spinal instability may continue unless surgically repaired.
- Most spinal fractures and surgical fusions heal in approximately 10 to 12 weeks.

Helpful Hints

- Surgical spinal instrumentation provides stabilization during healing, but the hardware will fail if bony fusion does not occur.
- Early surgical stabilization allows earlier mobilization and more intensive rehabilitation and results in shorter hospital length of stay.
- Quality of surgical stabilization, as judged by the surgeon, determines the need for external orthotic support.

Suggested Reading

Capagnolo DI, Heary RF. Acute medical and surgical management of spinal cord injury. In: Kirshblum S, Capagnolo DI, DeLisa JA, eds. *Spinal Cord Medicine*. Philadelphia: Lippincott Williams & Wilkins; 2002:96–107.

Section I: Conditions

Syndromes: Anterior Cord

Kemesha L. Delisser MD

Description
A lesion that affects the anterior two-thirds of the spinal cord, sparing the posterior columns, presenting as paralysis and hypoalgesia below the level of the lesion with preservation of touch, two-point discrimination, and vibratory sense.

Etiology/Types
- Hypoperfusion (65%)
- Spinal stenosis (25%)
- Trauma (12%)
- Disk compression
- Syphilitic arteritis
- Polyarteritis nodosa

Epidemiology
- Occurs in 2.7% of all traumatic SCIs
- Occurs in 1.2% of CNS vascular pathology

Pathogenesis
- The anterior two-thirds of the spinal cord includes the anterior horn cells (LMN) and the axons of the corticospinal (UMN) and spinothalamic tracts (pain, temperature).
- Damage occurs via mechanical compression or anterior spinal artery vascular insufficiency.
- Spinal cord infarction often occurs at vascular watershed areas around T1–T4 and L1, but may occur anywhere along cord.
- Central necrosis of spinal cord with gliosis and cavitation at the nerve root zones has been described as a common neuropathologic lesion with sparing of the dorsal columns.

Risk Factors
- Aortic or spinal surgery
- Hyperflexion injuries
- Arteriosclerotic disease
- Thrombotic disorder

Clinical Features
- Paralysis (LMN features usually predominate in cases due to hypoperfusion)
- Loss of pain and temperature perception
- Loss of bowel and bladder control

Natural History
- Symptoms typically progress rapidly.

Diagnosis

Differential diagnosis
- Transverse myelitis
- Guillain-Barre syndrome
- Tick paralysis
- Bilateral anterior cerebral artery occlusion

History
- Neurological symptoms following trauma/surgery
- Sudden neck or back pain
- Symmetric paralysis
- Decreased pain and temperature sensation

Exam
- Motor: weakness to level of lesion
- Sensory: pain and temperature loss below lesion, preservation of vibration and proprioception
- Reflexes: hyporeflexia or hyper-reflexia

Testing
- Spine X-rays, including flexion/extension views for stability evaluation
- MRI: for disk herniation, tumor, abscess, hematoma, infarct
- CT: for bony abnormalities
- Angiography, CTA/MRA: for vascular compromise
- Acetylneuraminic acid, RhF, anti-ds DNA if autoimmune disorder/vasculitis suspected

Pitfalls
- Intraoperative SSEPs primarily monitor posterior column pathways and may miss the presence of an anterior cord syndrome (ACS).

Red Flags
- Progression of paralysis
- Hemodynamic instability
- Fever (myelitis)

Treatment

Medical
- Directed at underlying cause, if known
- Airway protection if high cervical lesion

- Blood pressure support
- High-dose steroids may be beneficial in acute traumatic cases
- Nasogastric tube for paralytic ileus and gastric dilatation
- Bowel and bladder regimens
- Bracing and splinting as appropriate

Exercises
- Trunk balance and stabilization
- Neuromuscular facilitation exercises
- ADL and mobility training with attention to the use of appropriate assistive devices
- Body weight supported ambulation training

Modalities
- Functional electrical nerve stimulation for UMN paralysis

Injections
- Botulinum toxin for spasticity

Surgical
- Surgical decompression and spine stabilization for compressive causes
- Vascular repair in cases of arterial thrombus or dissection

Consults
- Physical medicine and rehabilitation
- Spine surgery
- Vascular surgery
- Neurology

Complications of treatment
- Infection

- Pain
- Worsening neurologic deficit
- Hardware loosening

Prognosis
- Prognosis generally poor and related to degree of neural damage
- When necrosis and hematomyelia occur, good outcome is unlikely even with surgery
- 10% to 20% chance of muscle recovery for all persons with ACS

Helpful Hints
- ACS can occur at any level of the spinal cord. If evidence of spared posterior column functions exist, ACS should be considered and evaluated for emergent treatment options (eg, surgery, steroids).
- Conventional MRI sequences will reveal ischemic lesions only after 10 to 15 hours from symptom onset. Diffusion-weighted imaging can identify ischemic lesions within a few minutes of clinical onset.

Suggested Readings
McKinley W, Santos K, Meade M, Brooke K. Incidence and outcomes of spinal cord injury clinical syndromes. *J Spinal Cord Med.* 2007;30:215–224.

Okamoto K, Hamada E, Okuda B. Anterior cerebral artery territory infarctions presenting with ascending tetraparesis. *J Stroke Cerebrovasc Dis.* 2004;13(2):92–94.

Sliwa JA, Maclean IC. Ischemic myelopathy: a review of spinal vasculature and related clinical syndromes. *Arch Phys Med Rehabil.* 1992;73(4):365–372.

Section I: Conditions

Syndromes: Brown-Séquard

Kemesha L. Delisser MD

Description
An incomplete lesion (hemisection) of the spinal cord that produces ipsilateral propioceptive and motor loss and contralateral loss of sensitivity to pain and temperature.

Etiology/Types
- Motor vehicle accidents (40%)
- Spinal stenosis (20%)
- Falls (13%)
- Tumor (13%)
- Gun shot wounds (7%)
- Spinal or epidural hematoma/abscess
- Cervical disk herniation (2% to 3%)
- Other penetrating injuries (eg, stabbing)

Epidemiology
- From 1% to 4% of all traumatic spinal cord injuries
- A hyperextension injury is the most common mechanism of injury.
- Brown-Séquard Plus syndrome or a partial Brown-Séquard syndrome (BSS) is more common and refers to a relative ipsilateral hemiplegia with a relative contralateral hemianalgesia.

Pathogenesis
- Degenerative changes, trauma, or compression damage on one side of the cord resulting in ipsilateral loss of motor function due to corticospinal tract compression at the level of the lesion combined with contralateral loss of pain and temperature sensation due to spinothalamic tract dysfunction.
- Spinothalamic tracts enter the cord and travel ipsilaterally for a few levels before crossing over; therefore, contralateral anesthesia usually begins one or two levels below the site of the lesion.
- Horner's syndrome may be present and is attributed to the involvement of ipsilateral descending sympathetic fibers within the cervical spinal cord.

Risk Factors
- Trauma especially to the cervical spine
- Spinal/epidural procedures
- Acceleration-deceleration events (MVA, roller coaster)

Clinical Features
- Hemiplegia with contralateral sensory loss
- Variable bladder/bowel dysfunction
- Depending on etiology, may have back/neck pain

Natural History
- Dependent on etiology and comorbidities
- Recovery typically takes place first in the proximal extensors followed by the distal flexors
- Most persons with BSS will regain mobility

Diagnosis

Differential diagnosis
- Multiple sclerosis
- Syringomyelia
- Spinal tumors

History
- Trauma
- Neck or back pain at level of lesion
- Recent spinal or epidural procedure

Exam
- Motor: ipsilateral weakness at level of lesion
- Sensory: ipsilateral loss of proprioception, vibration, and touch below lesion. Contralateral loss of pain and temperature below lesion
- Reflexes: ipsilateral hyporeflexia at level of lesion. Contralateral hyper-reflexia below lesion

Testing
- Abnormal findings on imaging typically are found more on one side than the other
- X-rays may demonstrate stenosis or fracture
- MRI: hyperintensity in a T2-weighted image representing traumatized cord; disk prolapse, abscess; tumor; or hematoma
- CT: osteophytes, displaced fractures, hematoma
- SSEPs may be used to demonstrate ipsilateral dorsal column involvement

Pitfalls
- Fall can be a cause or a consequence of BSS, so remember to search for antecedent trauma.

Red Flags
- History of other neurological deficits (think MS)

Treatment

Medical
- Treatment for individuals with BSS focuses on the underlying cause of the disorder.
- Early treatment with high-dose steroids may be beneficial.
- Other treatment is symptomatic and supportive.

Exercises
- Strengthening of weak muscles
- Body weight supported ambulation training

Modalities
- FES

Surgical
- Removal of foreign objects or spinal decompression surgery as indicated

Consults
- Physical medicine and rehabilitation
- Spine surgery
- Neurology

Complications
- Postoperative pain
- Pneumonia

Prognosis
- Best prognosis for ambulation of the SCI clinical syndromes.
- The extent to which a person recovers depends on the cause of injury and secondary conditions or complications.
- From 75% to 90% ambulate independently at discharge from rehabilitation.
- Nearly 70% perform functional skills and activities of daily living independently.

Helpful Hints
- A stronger lower limb increases the likelihood of ambulation at discharge.

Suggested Readings

McKinley W, Santos K, Meade M, Brooke K. Incidence and outcomes of spinal cord injury clinical syndromes. *J Spinal Cord Med.* 2007;30(3):215–224.

Roth EJ, Park T, Pang T, Yarkony GM, Lee MY. Traumatic cervical Brown-Sequard and Brown-Sequard-plus syndromes: The spectrum of presentations and outcomes. *Paraplegia.* 1991;29(9):582–589.

Tattersall R, Turner B. Brown-Sequard and his syndrome. *Lancet.* 2000;356(9223):61–63.

Section I: Conditions

Syndromes: Cauda Equina

Kemesha L. Delisser MD

Description
Cauda equina syndrome (CES) is an injury to the lumbo-sacral nerve roots within the neural canal.

Etiology/Types
- Trauma (40% to 45%)
- Spinal stenosis (25% to 30%)
- Tumor (10% to 15%)
- Infection (7%)
- Ischemia (2%)
- Sarcoidosis

Epidemiology
- From 1% to 6% of all lumbar disk herniations
- 5% of all SCIs

Pathogenesis
- An injury to the cauda equina, a bundle-like structure of nerve roots that extend caudally from the spinal cord, results in a LMN lesion.
- The cauda equina has only one layer of surrounding connective tissue, the endoneurium, making it more susceptible to injury.
- Region of relative hypovascularity below the conus may be more susceptible to ischemia.

Risk Factors
- Back injury
- Epidural anesthesia

Clinical Features
- Typically asymmetric but may be bilateral
- Low back pain
- Sciatica
- Sensory loss in root distribution
- Lower extremity weakness that may progress to paraplegia
- Weakness is LMN type (flaccid)
- Bowel and bladder dysfunction
- Erectile dysfunction

Natural History
- Can be an acute process or a slowly progressive condition, based on etiology
- Persistent pain
- UTIs

Diagnosis

Differential diagnosis
- Guillain-Barre syndrome
- Conus Medullaris syndrome
- Lumbosacral plexopathy
- Peripheral neuropathy
- Arachnoiditis
- Cytomegalovirus (CMV) or herpes simplex virus (HSV) infection in AIDS patients

History
- Low back pain
- Lower extremity weakness and/or radicular pain
- Urinary incontinence or retention
- Bowel incontinence or constipation
- Impotence

Exam
- Motor: weakness of anterior tibialis (L4, L5, S1), extensor hallucis longus (L4, L5, S1), hamstrings (L5, S1), gluteal muscles (L5, S1), gastrocnemius (L5, S1, S2) and decreased rectal tone (S2–S4). Atrophy of thigh or leg can be present in long standing disease
- Sensory: decreased perineal sensation (saddle anesthesia)
- Reflexes: impairment of bulbocavernous, plantar, and achilles tendon reflexes

Testing
- Urinalysis, HbA1c (to rule out other causes of bladder dysfunction)
- Lumbosacral spine X-rays, including flexion/extension views
- MRI: for disk herniation, tumor, abscess
- CT: for bony abnormalities
- Urodynamic studies
- Nerve conduction velocities (NCVs) are useful for differentiating peripheral neuropathy from radiculopathy.
- SSEPs are usually normal because the spinal nerve roots are compressed proximally to their dorsal root ganglions.

Pitfalls
- Urinary retention may occur initially, and then develop into overflow incontinence so someone may deny urinary incontinence but have high postvoid residual volumes.

Red Flags

- UMN signs [conus medullaris syndrome (CMS)]
- Fever (myelitis)
- Progression of paralysis

Treatment

Medical

- Treatment directed at the underlying cause
- High-dose steroids may be efficacious in acute traumatic setting.
- Intermittent catheterization and manual bowel program may be needed.
- Floor reaction type ankle foot orthoses are useful in the setting of plantar flexion weakness.

Exercises

- Strengthening, stretching, and ROM activities
- Neuromuscular facilitation exercises
- Body weight supported ambulation training

Surgical

- Surgical decompression and spine stabilization, if necessary
- Dorsal column stimulators may be indicated for chronic, severe pain.

Consults

- Physical medicine and rehabilitation
- Spine surgery
- Neurology

Complications of treatment

- Postoperative pain

- Pneumonia
- Wound infection
- Spinal fluid leak
- Epidural fibrosis

Prognosis

- Two thirds of persons either stabilize or improve after surgery, though wide variability exists.
- The extent of saddle sensory deficit is the most important predictor of recovery.
- People with complete perineal anesthesia are more likely to have permanent paralysis of the bladder.
- People with pain in both legs (bilateral sciatica) have less chance of full recovery than persons with single leg pain (unilateral sciatica).
- No good studies comparing surgery to conservative measures.

Helpful Hints

- Can present similarly to CMS, but CES is considered a pure lower motor lesion with absence of UMN signs.

Suggested Readings

Kennedy JG, Soffe KE, McGrath A, Stephens MM, Walsh MG, McManus F. Predictors of outcome in cauda equina syndrome. *Eur Spine J.* 1999;8(4):317–322.

Parke WW, Gammell K, Rothman RH. Arterial vascularization of the cauda equina. *J Bone Joint Surg Am.* 1981;63:53–56.

Spector LR, Madigan L, Rhyne A, Darden B, II, Kim D. Cauda equina syndrome. *J Am Acad Orthop Surg.* 2008;16:471–479.

Section I: Conditions

Syndromes: Central Cord

Danielle Perret MD

Description
A syndrome caused by a spinal cord lesion in the center of the cord, resulting in weakness greater in the upper extremities than lower extremities, bladder dysfunction, and varying sensory loss below the lesion.

Etiology/Types
- Falls and MVAs are the most common causes.
- Cervical stenosis with extension injury
- Major trauma, with fracture dislocation or compression fracture injuries
- Intramedullary hematoma, mass or syrinx, and rarely, cervical epidural abscess

Epidemiology
- Most common of the SCI syndromes, nearly 50%
- 9% of all traumatic SCIs
- Classically affects older persons with cervical spondylosis and a hyperextension injury
- C4–C5 is the most common level of injury.

Pathogenesis
- In hyperextension injury, anterior osteophytes or posterior infolded ligamentum flavum compress the cord.
- In fracture-dislocation or compression fracture, anterior-posterior forces compress the center of the cord.

Risk Factors
- Older age
- Cervical spondylosis or cervical spinal stenosis
- Hyperextension, acceleration-deceleration injury, fracture dislocation, or compression fracture of cervical spine

Clinical Features
- Greater weakness in arms than legs
- Sacral sensory sparing
- Bladder dysfunction
- Variations in sensory loss below the injury
- AIS "D" is the most common impairment score

Natural History
- Lower extremities recover first and to a greater extent.

- Proximal upper extremity recovery is greater than distal upper extremity recovery, with intrinsic hand muscles usually last

Diagnosis
Differential diagnosis
- Expanding intramedullary hematoma
- Syrinx

History
- Neurologic symptoms following trauma
- Neck pain
- Greater arm than leg weakness
- Urinary complaints
- Variable sensory complaints

Exam
- Perform ASIA examination; carefully assess spine.
- Perform general, physical, and neurologic examinations.

Testing
- CT of the cervical spine to assess the spinal column and associated fractures in acute injury
- MRI of the cervical spine to assess the spinal cord parenchyma, including evaluation for osseous injury, hemorrhage, and level of injury, which is identified by hyperintense signal
- Plain radiographs do not rule out central cord syndrome

Pitfalls
- Not excluded by normal imaging

Red Flags
- T2-weighted MRI signal intensity possible indicator of instability following a hyperextension injury

Treatment
Medical
- Acute traumatic SCI: consider high-dose methylprednisolone

Exercises
- Strengthening
- ROM

- Trunk balance and stabilization
- ADL and mobility training with attention to the use of appropriate assistive devices

Modalities
- Splinting, especially of the hands
- EMG biofeedback can be used to isolate specific muscles

Surgical
- Decompression and/or spinal stabilization if clinically indicated early: for persistent cord impingement, progression of neurologic deficits, or instability

Consults
- Physical medicine and rehabilitation
- Spine surgery

Complications of treatment
- Infection
- Pain below level of injury
- Hardware loosening
- Worsening neurologic function

Prognosis
- Favorable prognosis for functional recovery
- Prognosis is better for patients under age 50.

- Favorable prognostic factors include: good hand function, evidence of early motor recovery, young age, absence of spasticity
- Life expectancy depends on neurologic level, AIS, general health, medical and nursing care, and social support.
- Functional performance depends on neurological level, AIS, and general health.

Helpful Hints
- Poor trunk balance can limit ambulatory potential and the ultimate level of independence in many who have functional leg strength.

Suggested Readings
McKinley W, Santos K, Meade M, Brooke K. Incidence and outcomes of spinal cord injury clinical syndromes. *J Spinal Cord Med.* 2007;30:215–224.

Roth EJ, Lawler MH, Yarkony GM. Traumatic central cord syndromes: Clinical features and functional outcomes. *Arch Phys Med Rehabil.* 1990;71:18–23.

Song J, Mizuno J, Inoue T, Nakagawa H. Clinical evaluation of traumatic central cord syndrome: Emphasis on clinical significance of prevertebral hyperintensity, cord compression, and intramedullary high-signal intensity on magnetic resonance imaging. *Surg Neurol.* 2006;65(2):117–123.

Yamazaki T, Yanaka K, Fujita K, Kamezaki T, Uemura K, Nose T. Traumatic central cord syndrome: Analysis of factors affecting the outcome. *Surg Neurol.* 2005;63(2):95–99.

Section I: Conditions

Syndromes: Conus Medullaris

Kemesha L. Delisser MD

Description
Conus medullaris is an injury to the most distal region of the spinal cord (conus).

Etiology/Types
- Trauma (50% to 75%)
- Tumors (7%)
- Hypoperfusion (7%)
- Spinal stenosis (1%)
- Schistosomiasis
- Spinal cord tethering

Epidemiology
- From 1% to 2% of all spinal cord injuries

Pathogenesis
- The conus contains sacral spinal cord segments.
- Neurological deficits are typically caused by direct compression or ischemic injury.
- Since the conus is a small structure, a lesion involving it usually gives rise to bilateral signs.

Risk Factors
- Back injury
- Epidural anesthesia

Clinical Features
- Typically bilateral but may be asymmetric
- Low back pain, but may be painless
- Sciatica
- Saddle anesthesia
- Variable degrees of lower extremity weakness
- Bowel and bladder areflexia
- Erectile dysfunction

Natural History
- Can be an acute process or a slowly progressive condition, based on etiology

Diagnosis

Differential diagnosis
- CES
- Mixed conus medullaris syndrome/CES
- Diabetic neuropathy/plexopathy
- Parasitic infection
- Transverse myelitis

History
- Low back pain
- "Not feeling toilet tissue"
- Urinary incontinence or retention
- Bowel incontinence or constipation
- Impotence

Exam
- Motor: usually normal lower extremity motor function (LE). If S1/S2 involved, weakness of gastrocnemius, hamstrings, and gluteal muscles can be seen. Normal or decreased anal sphincter tone
- Sensory: decreased perineal sensation
- Reflexes: loss of bulbocavernous and achilles tendon reflexes. Patellar reflex is usually spared.
- Subacute lesions may produce upper motor neuron signs—hyper-reflexia, increased anal tone, and spastic bladder.

Testing
- Lumbosacral spine X-rays, including flexion/extension views
- MRI: for disk herniation, tumor, abscess
- CT: for bony abnormalities
- Urodynamic studies
- Electrodiagnostic studies can be useful for differentiating from peripheral neuropathy or radiculopathy.

Pitfalls
- Urinary retention often occurs initially developing into overflow incontinence, later creating a false impression of bladder recovery.

Red Flags
- Fever (myelitis)
- Progression of paralysis

Treatment

Medical
- Therapy generally directed at the underlying cause
- High-dose steroids may be efficacious in acute traumatic setting.
- Radiation for tumors

- Intermittent catheterization and manual bowel program may be needed.
- Teaching of Credé and Valsalva maneuvers to facilitate bladder emptying if areflexic
- Ankle foot orthoses

Exercises
- Strengthening, stretching, and ROM activities
- Gait training with assistive devices as needed

Surgical
- Spinal decompression and stabilization if indicated
- Dorsal column stimulators may be helpful for chronic, severe pain.
- Penile implants in cases of persistent erectile dysfunction

Consults
- Physical medicine and rehabilitation
- Spine surgery
- Neurology

Complications of treatment
- Postoperative pain
- Wound infection

Prognosis
- Traumatic lesions generally have poorer prognosis.
- At 1 month postinjury, a lower extremity motor score (LEMS) >10 signifies a high likelihood of community ambulation. LEMS is the sum of the lower extremity motor grades for the hip flexors, knee extensors, ankle dorsiflexors, great toe extensors, and ankle plantar flexors.
- People with complete perineal anesthesia are more likely to have permanent paralysis of the bladder.
- Presence of bulbocavernous reflex is associated with favorable prognosis of bladder function recovery.

Helpful Hints
- CMS can be present in the absence of any LE weakness.

Suggested Readings
Harrop JS, Hunt GE, Jr, Vaccaro AR. Conus medullaris and cauda equina syndrome as a result of traumatic injuries: management principles 1. *Neurosurg FOCUS.* 2004;16(6):1–23.

McKinley W, Santos K, Meade M, Brooke K. Incidence and outcomes of spinal cord injury clinical syndromes. *J Spinal Cord Med.* 2007;30(3):215–224.

Section I: Conditions

Syndromes: Posterior Cord

Danielle Perret MD

Description
Posterior cord syndrome is a selective injury to the posterior columns of the spinal cord presenting as loss of vibration sensation and proprioception below the level of the injury.

Etiology/Types
- Nontraumatic etiologies are most common
- Posterior spinal artery occlusion or infarcts
- Tumors
- Degenerative disc disease
- Vitamin B_{12} deficiency
- Traumatic etiologies include cervical hyperextension injuries

Epidemiology
- Least common of the SCI syndromes
- Incidence is <1%

Pathogenesis
- Direct compression injury to the posterior columns
- Vascular occlusion or infarction of the paired posterior spinal arteries (which provide blood to the posterior third of the spinal cord)

Risk Factors
- Hyperextension type injury
- Vitamin B_{12} deficiency
- Tumors
- Degenerative disc disease
- Risks for endovascular occlusion: syphilitic arteritis, cholesterol emboli from atheromatous aortic plaques, intrathecal injection of phenol, vertebral artery dissection, plasmocytoma

Clinical Features
- The majority of posterior spinal artery infarcts occur at the thoracolumbar level, although they have been observed in the cervical and thoracic levels.
- Loss of proprioception and vibration sense below the level of injury with preservation of muscle strength and pain and temperature sensation
- AIS "D" (motor incomplete) is the most frequent impairment classification.
- Wide-based or unsteady gait
- Coordination difficulties
- Painful paresthesias may be present.

Natural History
- Tend to have a favorable prognosis
- Neurologic recovery correlates in part to ASIA score
- Functional performance depends on neurologic level, AIS, and general health.
- Life expectancy depends on neurologic level, AIS, general health, medical and nursing care, and social support.
- Show the highest levels of control and independence during acute inpatient rehabilitation when compared to other SCI syndromes
- Progressive degeneration of the joints may occur.
- Charcot spine may occur.

Diagnosis

Differential diagnosis
- Myelitis due to infection or collagen disease
- Multiple sclerosis
- Polyneuropathy
- Tabes dorsalis
- Paraneoplasm

History
- Sudden or delayed onset of neurological symptoms below a given neurological level
- Vibration and proprioception sensory loss below the level of the lesion
- No loss of consciousness or cognitive deficits in absence of head injury

Exam
- Perform general, physical, and neurologic examinations.
- Perform ASIA motor and sensory exam to determine neurological level and degree of neurologic impairment.

Testing
- Laboratory test for B_{12} level, Venereal Disease Research laboratory test, Rapid Plasma Reagin test, or fluorescent treponemal antibody-absorption test may be warranted.
- X-rays may show no skeletal abnormality.
- CT may demonstrate skeletal injury.

- MRI findings may demonstrate disc disease or tumor with posterior cord impingement.
- MRI signal and enhancement features of spinal cord infarct may be nonspecific and can be seen in other diseases, such as multiple sclerosis and infectious myelitis.
- MRI findings should be complemented by blood and CSF laboratory data, brain MR imaging, and follow-up imaging of the spinal cord lesion.

Pitfalls

- Normal imaging studies do not exclude SCI.

Treatment

Medical

- Acute traumatic SCI: high-dose methylprednisolone for 24 to 48 hours can be considered.
- Other medications as appropriate for symptoms and signs
- Neuropathic pain medications (ie, antiepileptics) may be appropriate.

Exercises

- Trunk balance and stabilization
- Frankel exercises for ataxia
- Gait training, usually beginning in parallel bars
- Training in ADL, ambulation, and wheelchair mobility
- Joint proprioception exercises
- Upper extremity co-ordination exercises (Coulter exercises)
- Balance board

Surgical

- Usually not indicated
- Decompression and/or spinal stabilization if clinically indicated early: for persistent cord impingement, progression of neurologic deficits, or instability

Consults

- Physical medicine and rehabilitation
- Spine surgery

Complications of treatment

- Pain
- Progressive neurological decline
- Hardware loosening
- Infection
- Death

Prognosis

- Generally has a favorable prognosis for functional recovery

Helpful Hints

- Treat pain early

Suggested Readings

Kessler HH. *The Principles and Practices of Rehabilitation.* Manchester: Ayer, 1980:319.

Mascalchi M, Cosottini M, Ferrito G, Salvi F, Nencini P, Quilici N. Posterior spinal artery infarct. *Am J Neuroradiol.* 1998;19:361–363.

McKinley W, Santos K, Meade M, Brooke K. Incidence and outcomes of spinal cord injury clinical syndromes. *J Spinal Cord Med.* 2007;30:215–224.

Section I: Conditions

Syringomyelia and Tethered Cord

Harshpal Singh MD ■ Tanvir F. Choudhri MD

Description
Late neurologic decline can be seen after SCI and is frequently related to development of syrinx or tethered cord.

Etiology
- Syringomyelia
  - Cavitation of the spinal cord from direct cord injury
  - Cystic regions in prior cord hematoma
- Tethered cord
  - Scarring or adhesions between cord and spinal canal
- Syringomyelia and tethered cord may be inter-related processes.

Epidemiology
- Occurs in 21% to 28% of all spinal cord injuries
- From 1% to 9% of persons become symptomatic

Pathogenesis
- Syringomyelia
  - There is no consensus on the mechanism of post-traumatic syrinx formation.
  - Recent theory suggests syrinx results from repetitive mechanical distension of the spinal cord with subsequent accumulation of extracellular fluid within the distended cord (intramedullary pulse pressure theory).
  - Commonly found in watershed regions of the cord
- Tethered cord
  - Inflammation-induced scar or adhesion

Risk Factors
- Intraparenchymal cord hematoma

Clinical Features
- Develops 3 months to many years after injury
- Segmental dissociated sensory loss; more common than total sensory loss
- Segmental pain that is of a burning, dull, or aching quality, reflecting injury to spinothalamic pathways
- Pain exacerbated by coughing, sneezing, sitting, or straining
- Progressive asymmetrical weakness
- Asymmetric reduction in reflexes, hyperhidrosis, autonomic dysreflexia, Horner's syndrome

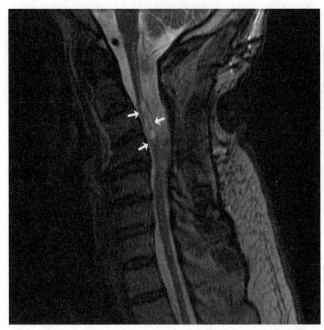

Syrinx. A syrinx in the cervical spinal cord is outlined by the arrows.

- Cardiopulmonary dysfunction
- Bulbar signs and symptoms if syrinx extends into brain stem

Natural History
- Most people demonstrate a slow progression of symptoms.
- Rapid progression in those that develop hemorrhage into syrinx from vessels in the cavity wall.
- Reports of spontaneous resolution in some people (thought to result from decompression of syrinx into subarachnoid space)

Diagnosis

Differential diagnosis
- Radiculopathy
- Spinal instability
- Canal stenosis

History
- New onset sensory deficit or segmental pain
- New onset motor weakness
- Increasing spasticity
- Gait changes

Exam
- Loss of pain and temperature with preservation of light touch and proprioception
- New onset hemiparesis
- Urinary incontinence
- Fecal incontinence
- LMN or UMN findings

Testing
- CT myelography
- Magnetic resonance imaging

Pitfalls
- Progressive enlargement with related mass effect on functional cord may result in irreversible neurologic deficit.

Red Flags
- New neurologic symptoms and signs
- New neuropathic pain

Treatment

Surgical
- Correction of deformity or compression
- Shunting
- Arachnolysis with or without duraplasty
- Cordectomy (rare)

Consults
- Neurologic spine surgery

Complications of treatment
- Persistent syrinx
- Worsening neurologic status
- Infection

Prognosis
- With appropriate treatment, stopping the progression of symptoms/deficits is generally possible.
- Improvement of symptoms and function is frequently possible, especially if detected/treated early.

Helpful Hints
- Dynamic MRI (with flexion/extension views) and MRI CSF flow studies can be helpful in assessing the presence and extent of cord tethering and syringomyelia.

Suggested Readings
Brodbelt AR, Stoodley MA. Post traumatic syringomyelia: A review. *J Clin Neurosci.* 2003;10(4):401–408.
Schurch B, Wichmann W, Rossier AB. Post-traumatic syringomyelia (cystic myelopathy): A prospective study of 449 patients with spinal cord injury. *J Neurol Neurosurg Psychiatry.* 1996;60(1):61–67.

Section I: Conditions

Thromboembolic Disease

Silvia G. Geraci DO ■ Adam B. Stein MD

Description

Thromboembolism includes deep venous thrombosis (DVT) and pulmonary embolism (PE). These are common complications of SCI and leading causes of morbidity and mortality.

Etiology/Types

■ DVTs are thrombi that develop in the deep venous systems of the limbs.
■ PEs occur when DVT embolizes to the pulmonary arterial circulation.

Epidemiology

■ The incidence of DVT after acute SCI without prophylaxis is over 50%.
■ The incidence of PE is approximately 5%.
■ 80% of DVTs develop within 2 weeks of SCI.

Pathogenesis

■ Virchow's triad includes endothelial damage, venous stasis, and hypercoagulable state.
■ Venous stasis is a direct result of paralysis and immobility.
■ Transient hypercoagulable state develops after SCI

Risk Factors

■ Motor complete injuries
■ Persons with paraplegia have a greater incidence of DVT than persons with tetraplegia
■ The incidence of PE is unrelated to level or extent of injury
■ Males
■ Lower extremity fracture
■ History of thromboembolism
■ Cancer
■ Heart failure
■ Obesity
■ Age over 70 years
■ Pregnancy or estrogen therapy

Clinical Features

■ Limb pain, erythema, swelling for DVT
■ Tachycardia, tachypnea, dyspnea, chest pain, fever, and arrhythmia for PE

Natural History

■ DVTs can extend proximally and migrate to become PEs
■ Post-thrombotic syndrome includes chronic edema, pain, induration, and skin ulceration
■ Pulmonary edema, cor pulmonale

Diagnosis

Differential diagnosis

■ DVT: superficial phlebitis, cellulitis, fracture, heterotopic ossification, arterial occlusion
■ PE: pneumonia, myocardial infarction, pneumothorax

History

■ Pain in limb associated with swelling, though SCI patients are often asymptomatic.

Exam

■ Unilateral edema
■ Pain, tenderness, and/or erythema of limb
■ Low-grade fever
■ Tachycardia, tachypnea, cardiac arrhythmia

Testing

■ Doppler ultrasound of limb
■ Spiral CT of the lungs
■ Ventilation-perfusion scan
■ EKG changes in PE are characterized by a right ventricular strain pattern
■ Venogram and pulmonary angiogram are gold standards but are frequently unnecessary

Pitfalls

■ Persons with SCI with a DVT are frequently asymptomatic.
■ Doppler ultrasound has a lower sensitivity in asymptomatic patients.
■ Doppler ultrasound may not visualize all veins of the LE.
■ Ventilation-perfusion scan reports are often inconclusive.

Red Flags

■ Sudden onset of shortness of breath, chest pain, and hypoxia warrants an immediate evaluation for suspected PE.

Treatment

Medical

- DVT prophylaxis should begin within 72 hours of injury
- Prophylaxis should continue until time of discharge for motor incomplete SCI, for 8 weeks in uncomplicated complete injuries, and for 12 weeks in complete motor injuries with additional risk factors
- Low–molecular-weight heparin is indicated for prophylaxis
- Pneumatic compression is begun as soon as possible and continued for 2 weeks after SCI
- Compression stockings
- Duration of treatment for thromboemboli:
  - For a known DVT, anticoagulate 3 to 6 months
  - For a known PE, anticoagulate 6 months

Exercises

- Early mobilization
- Passive ROM

Surgical

- Vena cava filter is placed in patients who fail or have a contraindication to anticoagulation.
- Filters should be strongly considered for motor complete injuries with additional risk factors.

Consults

- Vascular surgery or interventional radiology for vena cava filter placement

Complications of treatment

- Filter migration or vena cava perforation
- Skin infections at site of entry of inferior vena cava filter
- Heparin-induced thrombocytopenia
- Bleeding related to anticoagulants
- Skin breakdown from compression stockings or pneumatic compression sleeves

Prognosis

- PE is third leading cause of death in SCI patients within 1 year of injury.

Helpful Hints

- If patient has known DVT or PE, hold mobilization and ROM for 48 to 72 hours while anticoagulation initiated.
- If surgery is necessary, hold anticoagulation the morning of the procedure and resume 1 day postoperatively.
- Initiate treatment of thrombus with both heparinoid and warfarin in patients with low bleeding risk.
- Routine noninvasive screening for DVT with Doppler ultrasound should be considered for all patients with SCI because of the frequency of occurrence and the frequent absence of clinical findings.
- Avoid phlebotomy and intravenous insertions in the legs of SCI patients to avoid endothelial injury.

Suggested Readings

Chen D. Thromboembolism in spinal cord disorders. In: Lin VW, Cardenas DD, et al., eds. *Spinal Cord Medicine Principles and Practice*. New York: Demos, 2003:193–207.

Consortium for spinal cord injury medicine et al. Prevention of thromboembolism in spinal cord injury. *J Spinal Cord Med*. 1997;20(3):259–283.

Section I: Conditions

Traumatic Brain Injury

Neil N. Jasey Jr. MD

Description

Traumatic brain injury (TBI) is defined as brain injury from externally inflicted trauma variably associated with alteration or loss of consciousness (LOC), abnormal Glasgow Coma Scale (GCS), presence of posttraumatic amnesia (PTA), and/or abnormal neuroimaging findings.

Etiology/Types

■ Mild
■ Mild complicated
■ Moderate
■ Severe
■ TBI classification is determined by the presence, absence, and/or duration of LOC, PTA, GCS abnormalities and neuroimaging findings

Epidemiology

■ TBI is estimated to occur in 16% to 74% of traumatic SCIs depending on method of identification for TBI.
■ TBI is more frequent in persons with tetraplegia than paraplegia.

Pathogenesis

■ Primary injury results from contusion and shear forces at impact
■ Key components of primary injury include cortical disruption, axonal injury, vascular damage, cerebral swelling/edema, and hemorrhage
■ Secondary injury results from hypotension, hypoxemia, and a cascade of events variably causing ischemia, excitotoxicity, energy failure, and cellular death
■ Axonal damage
■ Inflammation and regeneration

Risk Factors

■ Essentially identical to those for SCI

Clinical Features

■ Early symptoms of TBI include altered consciousness, cognition, and behavior, eg, various stages of coma, mental confusion, impaired memory, agitation, and disinhibition.
■ Late symptoms of TBI may include those of postconcussive syndrome, eg, headaches, dizziness, fatigue, irritability, emotional lability, impaired memory or ability to concentrate, and insomnia, or failure to progress during rehabilitation.

Natural History

■ Functional outcomes are predicted by severity of the TBI, the level and completeness of the SCI.
■ Symptoms of TBI tend to improve over time, but extent of recovery varies.
■ Late effects of TBI include reduced functional gains, increased healthcare costs, greater demand on clinician resources, substance abuse, and so on.

Diagnosis

Differential diagnosis

■ Side effects of medications, for example, tranquilizers, narcotics, steroids, and so on
■ Pre-existing conditions affecting cognition, mood, and behavior
■ Intensive care unit psychosis

History

■ Reported LOC, abnormal GCS, and/or presence of PTA
■ Altered consciousness, cognition, and behavior
■ High-level SCI caused by motor vehicle collision (MVC) or fall from height
■ Low cognitive functional independence measure (FIM) scores
■ Slow functional progress during rehabilitation

Exam

■ In acute TBI, exam focuses on identifying location, type, and magnitude of injury in order to select proper surgical and/or medical treatment.
■ In postacute TBI, exam includes assessment of neurologic, cognitive, and behavioral symptoms, eg, GCS, PTA, Rancho Los Amigos Level of Cognitive Function (RLALCF), memory, orientation, ability to follow directions, and symptoms that may affect functional progress.

Testing

■ Imaging of head/brain, ie, X-rays, CT, MRI
■ Assess persons GCS and perform minimental status exam

- Comprehensive neuropsychological evaluation in select cases

Pitfalls

- Failure to recognize TBI in persons with SCI may result in ineffective rehabilitation and lower than expected functional outcomes.

Red Flags

- Failure to progress during rehabilitation and/or to adjust in the community following high-level SCI caused by MVC or fall from heights may suggest concomitant TBI.

Treatment

Medical

- Neurostimulants to increase arousal and attention
- Antipsychotics to treat aggression and agitation
- Anticonvulsants to treat seizures, emotionalability, or agitation

Surgical

- Monitor intracranial pressure
- Evacuation of hematomas causing mass effect
- Cranioplasty for large bony defects

Consults

- Physical medicine and rehabilitation
- Neurosurgery
- Neurology
- Neuropsychology
- Psychiatry

Complications of treatment

- Infection after neurosurgical procedures
- Side effects from medications

Prognosis

- Worse outcomes after TBI are associated with older age, low initial GCS, long duration of PTA and coma, and severe damage shown on early neuroimaging.

Helpful Hints

- Suspect TBI in persons with high level neurologically complete SCI caused by high-velocity MVC or fall from heights, especially if person is not progressing well on rehabilitation program.

Suggested Readings

Ashley MJ, ed. *Traumatic Brain Injury:Rehabilitative Treatment and Case Management.* Boca Raton, FL: CRC Press, 2004.

Macciocchi S, Seel RT, Thompson N, Byams R, Bowman B. Spinal cord injury and co-occurring traumatic brain injury: assessment and incidence. *Arch Phys Med Rehabil.* 2008;89:1350–1357.

Macciocchi SN, Bowman B, Coker J, Apple D, Leslie D. Effect of comorbid traumatic brain injury on functional outcome of persons with spinal cord injuries. *Am J Phys Med Rehabil.* 2004;83:22–26.

Tolonen A, Turkka J, Salonen O, Ahoniemi E, Alaranta H. Traumatic brain injury is underdiagnosed in patients with spinal cord injury. *J Rehabil Med.* 2007;39: 622–626.

Zasler ND, Katz DI, Zafonte RD, eds. *Brain Injury Medicine: Principles and Practice.* New York: Demos, 2007.

Section I: Conditions

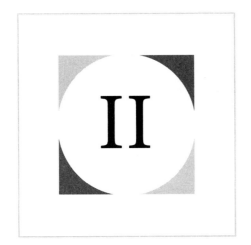

Interventions

Airway Management: Tracheostomy

Kenneth W. Altman MD PhD ■ Chih-Kwang Sung MD MS

Description

A tracheostomy is a tracheocutaneous fistula or a procedure that creates one.

Key Principles

- Perform emergently or electively by open surgical or percutaneous dilation techniques

Indications

- To bypass upper airway obstruction
- To assist respiration over prolonged periods
- To assist with pulmonary hygiene
- To manage aspiration of oral or gastric secretions
- After maxillofacial or laryngotracheal trauma

Relative Contraindications and Concerns

- Soft tissue infection of neck
- Anatomic abnormalities
- Coagulopathies
- Hemodynamic instability
- High positive pressure ventilation

Special Considerations

- Perform tracheostomy within 2 to10 days after intubation
- Perform tracheostomy in patients with traumatic brain injury presenting with Glascow Coma Score (GCS) ≤8 who are at risk for prolonged intubation >7 days
- A tracheostomy tube is less noxious for the patient emerging from coma than an endotracheal tube and sedation can be more easily weaned
- A tracheostomy can facilitate weaning from a ventilator by allowing progressive ventilator free breathing
- Usually does not interfere with oral food intake

Key Procedural Steps

Surgical tracheostomy

- Make a vertical or horizontal incision 1 cm below cricoid cartilage through the skin and platysma
- Separate the strap muscles in the midline
- Retract or divide the thyroid isthmus
- Make an incision into the trachea, usually between the second and third tracheal rings, with or without creation of Björk flap (incised tracheal ring sutured to skin)
- Alternatively, resect the tracheal ring or make a cruciate incision in trachea
- Insert the tracheostomy tube

Percutaneous dilational tracheostomy

- Make a small horizontal incision in the skin 1 cm below the cricoid cartilage
- Insert a needle transcutaneously into trachea, preferably with flexible bronchoscopic guidance to insure midline placement in tracheal ring and reduce posterior tracheal wall trauma
- Pass a guide wire into the tracheal lumen
- Serial dilate
- Insert the tracheostomy tube

Anticipated Problems

Early complications

- Hemorrhage
- Infection
- Subcutaneous emphysema
- Pneumothorax
- Pneumomediastinum
- Postoperative pulmonary edema
- Loss of airway; tube dislodgement
- Mucus plug

Late complications

- Granulation tissue
- Tracheal/subglottic stenosis
- Tracheal-innominate artery fistula
- Tracheoesophageal fistula
- Tracheocutaneous fistula

Helpful Hints

Tracheostomy tubes

- Always use the obturator for insertion of tube and remove immediately after insertion
- Tubes can be metal, plastic, or silicone and can be cuffed, uncuffed, or fenestrated
- Cuffed tubes have a balloon at the distal tip for inflation during mechanical ventilation
- Uncuffed tubes allow air to pass around the tube

- Fenestrated tubes have an opening that permits speech when the external opening is capped
- A speaking valve is a one-way valve that may be placed over the external opening to allow vocalization without blocking inspiratory airflow through the tube

Tracheostomy care

- Maintain tube with stay sutures and ties for at least 48 to 72 hours
- Humidification of air and gentle saline irrigation of mucus reduces likelihood of mucus plug or crust
- Maintain cuff pressure less than capillary pressure (<25 cm H_2O) to reduce likelihood of development of tracheal stenosis or malacia
- Apply stomal dressing to prevent skin breakdown
- Change tracheostomy tube only after tract has formed (after 3 to 5 days)
- Avoid solid food intake while cuff is inflated

Decannulation—removal of tube

- Confirm all indications for tracheostomy are resolved
- Remove tube as soon as possible to avoid late complications
- Serially downsize tube to a smaller, cuffless one
- Cap tube and only decannulate after at least 24 hours of continuous tube occlusion
- Consider flexible or other laryngoscopy if patient is unable to tolerate occlusion/capping of tube
- Place occlusive dressing over stoma after tube removal and change daily until stoma closes

Suggested Readings

Groves DS, Durbin CG, Jr. Tracheostomy in the critically ill: indications, timing and techniques. *Curr Opin Crit Care.* 2007;13(1):90–97.

Gurkin SA, Parikshak M, Kralovich KA, et al. Indicators for tracheostomy in patients with traumatic brain injury. *Am Surg.* 2002;68:324–328, discussion 8–9.

Major KM, Hui T, Wilson MT, et al. Objective indications for early tracheostomy after blunt head trauma. *Am J Surg.* 2003;186:615–619.

Section II: Interventions

Bladder Management: Indwelling Urinary Catheters

Adam B. Stein MD

Description

Indwelling catheters are one of the mainstays of urologic management in persons with SCI. Management with indwelling catheters may represent either a temporary strategy, or a long-term care plan. Types of indwelling catheters include transurethral catheters and suprapubic catheters, which enter the bladder directly through an incision in the lower abdominal wall.

Key Principles

Short-term use of indwelling urethral catheter

- A Foley catheter should be placed in the early phase of an acute SCI, when the primary goal is securing adequate urinary drainage while tending to the patients hemodynamic status, associated injuries, and spine stability.

Short-term use of suprapubic catheter

- A suprapubic cystostomy is indicated in the acute period after spinal trauma if there is associated urethral trauma that precludes placement of an indwelling urethral catheter.

Long-term use of indwelling urethral or suprapubic catheter

- Poor hand function
- High daily urine output
- High-pressure detrusor-sphincter dyssynergia
- Vesicoureteral reflux or hydronephrosis
- Inability to tolerate, or find success, with other less intrusive forms of bladder management such as intermittent catheterization or reflex voiding
- Limited caregiver assistance, making other methods of bladder management untenable

Long-term use of suprapubic catheter

- Urethral abnormalities (eg, stricture, false passage, hypospadias)
- Difficulty inserting urethral catheters
- Recurrent prostatitis or epididymitis
- The need for indwelling catheterization but a desire to decrease some potential risks of transurethral indwelling catheters such as traumatic hypospadias, prostatitis, and urethral false passage

- The need for indwelling catheterization, but a desire for greater sexual activity or enhanced body image than that allowed for by a transurethral catheter
- Recurrent indwelling urethral catheter obstruction at the level of the urethra (eg, intermittent spasticity of the external sphincter with obstruction to flow)

Contraindications

- Avoid suprapubic catheters when persistent incontinence is the result of an incompetent sphincter. In such cases, incontinence persists unless sphincter incompetence is treated.
- Urethral catheters should be avoided in pelvic trauma with suspected urethral injury. Indicators of urethropelvic trauma include blood at the urethral meatus and pelvic or scrotal hematomas.

Special Considerations

- Indwelling catheters are recommended for spinal cord injured individuals with significant cognitive impairment or active substance abuse.
- Suprapubic catheters are completely reversible should a different preferred method of bladder management be identified.

Key Procedural Steps

- At the time of spinal injury, place an indwelling urethral catheter unless urethropelvic trauma is suspected.
- Maintain indwelling catheter until the patient has entered the rehabilitation phase of treatment, is medically stable, and psychologically prepared for removal of the catheter.
- If persistent use of indwelling urethral catheter is indicated, change catheter every 2 to 4 weeks, unless there is a history of bladder stones or catheter encrustation, in which case catheter is changed every 1 to 2 weeks.
- For a suprapubic cystostomy, catheter change is every 4 weeks unless there is a history of bladder stone or catheter encrustation, in which case it is changed every 1 to 2 weeks. Insert a new catheter immediately upon removing old catheter to preserve the tract to the bladder.

- It is preferred that the catheter inserted be latex free to avoid development of latex allergy.
- For urethral catheters, 14 to 16 Fr is the preferred size. The balloon should contain 5 to 10 mL of water. For suprapubic catheters, the preferred catheter size is 22 to 24 Fr.

Anticipated Problems

- Urethral erosions can be avoided by anchoring catheter to abdomen with belt or tape
- Catheter clogging can be treated with gentle saline bladder irrigation or with instillation of Renacidin daily for 20 to 30 minutes
- Chronic indwelling catheters increase the risk for developing bladder cancer, necessitating surveillance that may include cytology, cystoscopy, and bladder biopsy
- Kidney and bladder stones
- Recurrent UTI
- Pyelonephritis
- Epididymitis
- Incontinence
- Hydronephrosis from bladder wall hypertrophy

Helpful Hints

- Adequate fluid intake facilitates mechanical washout of bladder debris, decreasing the likelihood of bladder stones.
- Anticholinergic agents can be helpful when used in the setting of indwelling catheters to maintain bladder capacity and decrease the risk of hydronephrosis, bladder contractions, and autonomic dysreflexia provoked by the catheter balloon.

Suggested Reading

Consortium for Spinal Cord Medicine et al. Clinical practice guideline: bladder management for adults with spinal cord injury. *J Spinal Cord Med*. 2006;29(5):527–573.

Section II: Interventions

Bladder Management: Intermittent Catheterization

Matthew M. Shatzer DO

Description

Intermittent catheterization (IC) is a method of emptying the bladder at specific time intervals by inserting a catheter into the bladder, draining the urine, and then removing the catheter. The intent is for the individual to be catheter-free between insertions.

Key Principles

- Do not begin IC until fluid resuscitation is complete and urine output is <2 L/24 h.
- IC should be performed frequently enough to prevent the bladder from becoming overdistended (<400 to 500 mL per insertion).
- IC is associated with a lower risk of hydronephrosis, bladder and renal calculi, autonomic dysreflexia, urethral incompetence, and erosions as compared to the use of indwelling catheters.
- Increase the frequency of intermittent catheterization or decrease fluid intake if catheterized volumes consistently exceed 500 mL.
- Individuals and their caregivers should be educated regarding clean technique before discharge from rehabilitation unit.
- IC is associated with a better self-image and enhanced sexual function when compared to other methods of management.
- Intermittent bladder filling that occurs with IC prevents the reduction of bladder capacity and compliance that is frequently seen in other methods of bladder management.

Indications

- Any individual with a spinal cord injury who has not recovered normal urination, has adequate hand function, or has a caregiver willing to perform catheterization

Contraindications

- Inadequate hand function or absence of a caregiver available to perform catheterization
- Abnormal urethral anatomy such as strictures, false passages, and bladder neck obstruction
- Bladder capacity <200 mL

- High fluid intake
- Poor cognition
- Inability or unwillingness to adhere to a regular schedule
- Adverse psychological reaction to IC
- Tendency to develop autonomic dysreflexia with bladder filling
- Severe adductor spasticity, particularly in women

Special Considerations

- Must regularly monitor the lower and upper urinary tracts for early signs of complications
- Most individuals can perform the clean, rather than sterile technique
- Consider sterile technique for persons with recurrent symptomatic UTI
- The frequency of catheterization is typically every 4 to 6 hours. If collected urine exceeds 500 mL, fluid intake should be reduced.

Key Procedural Steps

- Use a catheter that is easy to insert without trauma. Catheters of varying stiffness are available.
- Catheters can be cleaned with a mild soap and air-dried between uses if a new catheter is not available.
- In the case of recurrent UTIs, the individual's technique must be assessed.

Anticipated Problems

- Autonomic dysreflexia
- Overdistention in noncompliant patients
- UTI
- Urethral trauma with hematuria
- Urethral stricture or false passages
- Urinary tract stones

Helpful Hints

- If patient leaks urine between catheterizations, treatment with anticholinergic agent may be beneficial.
- Early education and training on rehabilitation unit is important.

Suggested Readings

Consortium for Spinal Cord Medicine et al. Bladder management for adults with spinal cord injury. *J Spinal Cord Med.* 2006;29(5):527–573.

Linsenmeyer TA. Neurogenic bladder following spinal cord injury. In: Kirshblum S, Campagnolo DI, DeLisa JA, eds. *Spinal Cord Medicine*. Philadelphia: Lippincott Williams & Wilkins; 2002:181–206.

Bladder Management: Sphincterotomy and Endourethral Stenting

Adam B. Stein MD

Description

Endourethral stenting and transurethral sphincterotomy are procedures used for spinal cord injured men with detrusor-sphincter dyssynergia (DSD) who void reflexively and are committed to wearing an external catheter.

Key Principles

- Endourethral stenting involves the deployment of a tubular metallic mesh stent at the level of the dyssynergic external sphincter.
- The stent maintains the sphincter in an open, nonobstructing position.
- The stent is placed transurethrally and is removable.
- Transurethral external sphincterotomy (TURES) is ideally performed with a Holmium contact laser.
- After stenting or TURES, the desired result is voiding pressure <40 cm H_2O.

Indications

- Unable or unwilling to perform intermittent catheterization
- Autonomic dysreflexia with reflex voiding
- Poor bladder drainage with reflex voiding with evidence of upper tract deterioration or the potential for upper tract deterioration

Contraindications

- Being female
- Inability to maintain a condom catheter due to small retracting penis, poor hand function, or lack of caregiver assistance
- Urethral structural abnormalities

Key Procedural Steps

Endourethral stent

- Preoperatively, decide upon type of anesthesia as those with a history of dysreflexia or severe spasticity should receive spinal or general anesthesia.
- Stent arrives preloaded on docking tool.
- Ideal placement of stent is such that proximal end extends to the distal end of the colliculus seminalis (to avoid blockage of the ejaculatory ducts) and the distal end of the stent rests in the bulbar urethra.

- Stent expands upon deployment to approximately 14 mm (42 Fr) and is maintained in place through its mesh configuration and elastic properties.
- Many urologists place a suprapubic tube at the time of stent placement until adequate stent function is demonstrated.
- In the postoperative period, care is taken to avoid stent migration including avoiding catheterization until epithelialization occurs.
- Individuals with a stent should be seen regularly to ensure desired stent function. Follow-up evaluation should include urodynamics and urethroscopy.

Transurethral external sphincterotomy

- The same anesthetic considerations apply to TURES as for stent.
- Laser is applied through a standard cystoscope and delivered fiber-optically.
- TURES usually extends from colliculus seminalis to the proximal bulbar urethra.
- Incision usually located at most superior aspect of the external sphincter.
- The resection should be full thickness, cutting all muscle fibers.
- Usually, repeated passes through sphincter are required.
- Postoperatively, the individual must be monitored for bleeding.
- Follow-up urodynamics are useful to ensure voiding pressures in desired range.

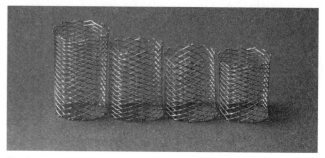

Endourethral stent (AMS Urolume Courtesy of American Medical Systems, Inc. Minnetonka, Minnesota, www.AmericanMedicalSystems.com).

Anticipated Problems

Endourethral stent

- Stent migration with need for repeat procedure
- Stone encrustation
- If stent removal is required, it may be technically difficult and traumatic
- Tissue hyperplasia at stent can result in obstructive uropathy
- Urethral pain and trauma

Transurethral external sphincterotomy

- Perioperative bleeding and clot retention
- Need for reoperation in substantial number of cases due to lack of desired effect
- Urethral stricture
- Erectile and ejaculatory dysfunction
- Decreased ability to be urine free during sexual activity

Helpful Hints

- Urethral stent placement is generally preferable to TURES because of its reported efficacy, potential reversibility, and minimal morbidity.
- Should indwelling catheters be required following successful stent or TURES, leakage around the catheter may occur.
- For the first 3 months following stent placement, consider altering transfer methods to minimize risk of stent migration, including use of a sliding board or a mechanical lift for persons with tetraplegia.

Suggested Readings

Chancellor MB, et al. Sphincteric stent versus external sphincterotomy in spinal cord injured men: prospective randomized multicenter trial. *J Urol.* 1999;161(6):1893–1898.

Consortium for Spinal Cord Medicine et al. Clinical practice guideline: bladder management for adults with spinal cord injury. *J Spinal Cord Med.* 2006;29(5):527–573.

Bladder Management: Urinary Diversion and Bladder Augmentation

Adam B. Stein MD

Description

Bladder augmentation, or augmentation cystoplasty, is a surgical procedure designed to allow successful intermittent catheterization and restoration of continence in the setting of persistent detrusor hyper-reflexia with incontinence. Urinary diversion procedures are used for spinal cord injured individuals who would benefit from diversion of urine away from the bladder. Diversion procedures include continent and standard (incontinent) diversions.

Key Principles

- Bladder augmentation improves bladder capacity and reduces intravesical pressure by incorporating a patch of intestinal tissue taken from ileum, colon, or stomach.
- Successful augmentation cystoplasty can restore continence between catheterizations and can eliminate reflux or hydronephrosis related to detrusor sphincter dyssynergia (DSD).
- Continent diversions, such as the Kock Pouch and the Indiana Pouch, create a neobladder with an associated continent stoma, often using the appendix to create the catheterizable stoma located at the umbilicus (Mitrofanoff procedure).
- The Mitrofanoff procedure may also be used in association with the patient's native bladder.
- An incontinent diversion, such as an ileovesicostomy, utilizes an intestinal segment to create a neobladder that is brought to the skin of the abdominal wall. Urine drains to an external collecting bag.

Indications

Augmentation cystoplasty

- Individuals with the desire to perform intermittent catheterization (IC) but are incontinent because of uncontrollable bladder contractions despite medical therapy
- Individuals at high risk for renal damage in the setting of reflux or hydronephrosis resulting from DSD

Continent urinary diversion

- Persons unable to easily access their urethra for IC because of spasticity, contracture, obesity, or limited hand function in tetraplegia
- Individuals who have an incompetent bladder outlet, urethral erosions, or fistulas or severe pressure ulcers negatively affected by incontinence
- Persons who require cystectomy (eg, bladder cancer)

Incontinent diversion

- Persons requiring a diverting procedure for the reasons listed above, but who do not have the hand function necessary to utilize a catheterizable stoma

Contraindications

- Inflammatory bowel disease
- Pelvic irradiation
- Abdominal adhesions
- Poor kidney function

Special Considerations

- Augmentation cystoplasty may be combined with procedures to provide a catheterizable stoma (eg, Mitrofanoff) or to improve an incompetent outlet (eg, sling procedure). Ideally, this should be performed as a single procedure.

Key Procedural Steps

Preoperative

- Bowel preparation/cleansing for intestinal harvesting; provide low residue diet
- Determination of stoma location; patient should be evaluated in supine and sitting. Stoma should not be placed at belt line of clothing

Perioperative

- Nasogastric tube may be placed until bowel function returns.
- Placement of suprapubic tube and Foley catheter for bladder augmentation to protect bladder-intestinal anastamosis until healed.

Postoperative

- Irrigate bladder with normal saline to clear mucus secreted by intestinal segment
- Monitor electrolytes for potential hyperchloremic metabolic acidosis

Anticipated Problems

- Postoperative ileus
- Small bowel obstruction
- Excessive mucus production that can clog catheter and obstruct drainage
- Disruption to bowel routine, usually self-corrects in first month
- Dehiscence of surgical anastamosis
- Hyperchloremic metabolic acidosis
- Vitamin B_{12} deficiency

- Stomal stenosis with difficulty catheterizing

Helpful Hints

- It is useful to have the patient demonstrate the anticipated necessary care preoperatively, including intermittent catheterization or application of an external collecting device.

Suggested Readings

Consortium for Spinal Cord Medicine et al. Clinical practice guideline: bladder management for adults with spinal cord injury. *J Spinal Cord Med.* 2006;29(5):527–573.

Linsenmeyer TA. Neurogenic bladder following spinal cord injury. In: Kirshblum S, Campagnolo DI, DeLisa JA, eds. *Spinal Cord Medicine.* Philadelphia: Lippincott, Williams & Wilkins; 2002:181–206.

Bladder Management: Urodynamic Testing

Matthew M. Shatzer DO

Description

Urodynamic testing is a physiologic diagnostic study of the lower urinary tract. It is a method of studying normal and abnormal physiology related to the storage, transport, and emptying of urine from the bladder. It provides information about bladder and sphincter function.

Key Principles

- Urodynamic testing measures the storage and emptying or voiding phases.
- A complete urodynamic test will include a cystometrogram (CMG), sphincter EMG, uroflowmetry, pressure flow evaluation, and postvoid residual determination.
- CMG is a tool used to evaluate the storage phase of micturition.
- During CMG the bladder is filled through a catheter, with either CO_2 or water, and intravesical pressures are measured.
- CMG provides information on the compliance, stability, and capacity of the bladder.
- Water is preferred as a filling medium as it is more physiologic than gas.
- Sphincter EMG monitors relaxation and contraction of the external sphincter muscle during the course of bladder filling and emptying.
- In an individual with detrusor-sphincter dysynergia (DSD), sphincter EMG activity increases during bladder contraction creating a functional obstruction to flow.
- Uroflowmetry measures the speed of urinary flow.
- At the completion of emptying, a postvoid residual volume is recorded.
- Videourodynamics is an advanced study that involves the measurement of bladder, abdominal, and sphincter pressures while fluoroscopically imaging the bladder.

Indications

- Urodynamic studies are indicated in most spinal cord injured individuals to assess voiding function.
- Videourodynamics are indicated for the evaluation of
  - Presence and severity of DSD
  - Presence of mechanical obstruction
  - Efficacy of pharmacotherapy
  - Suitability for a potential surgical procedure
  - Individuals with recurrent UTIs.

Contraindications

- Active UTI
- Allergy to contrast dye (videourodynamics)

Special Considerations

- Monitor closely for autonomic dysreflexia during exam in individuals with neurological levels above T6

Key Procedural Steps

- A two-channel catheter is used during CMG; one for filling bladder, the other for measuring pressures.
- The typical bladder filling rate is 25 to 60 mL of H_2O/min
- During bladder filling, the individual is asked to suppress voiding.
- In the filling phase, bladder sensation is recorded and bladder capacity, wall compliance, and stability are measured.
- The normal individual typically describes the first sensation of bladder fullness at 100 to 200 mL, and the sensation of urgency between 400 and 500 mL.
- During the voiding phase, pressure at which voiding begins is measured, as is flow rate, sphincter EMG activity, voided volume, and postvoid residual volume.

Anticipated Problems

- Autonomic dysreflexia
- UTI
- Results of urodynamic testing are not always representative of the individual's clinical status, for example, an intact individual may have difficulty voiding in the urodynamic lab.

Helpful Hints

- The clinician should attempt to perform the study and position of the individual in such a way as to make the filling and voiding phases as natural as possible, for example, an individual who typically voids while sitting should be tested in a seated position.

- Bladder compliance is defined as the change in volume/increase in baseline pressure.
- Compliance should be greater than 10 mL/cm H_2O.
- Sphincter EMG does not identify individual motor units, and is therefore only useful in determining the contraction and relaxation of the sphincter.
- Abdominal pressure tracings determine if person is using the abdominal musculature to assist with voiding as opposed to relying solely on contraction of the detrusor.

Suggested Readings

Cardenas DD, Mayo ME. Management in bladder dysfunction. In: Braddom RL, ed. *Physical Medicine and Rehabilitation.* 3rd ed. Philadelphia : Elsevier; 2007:621–624.

Consortium for Spinal Cord Medicine et al. Clinical practice guideline: bladder management for adults with spinal cord injury. *J Spinal Cord Med.* 2006;29(5):527–573.

Linsenmeyer TA. Neurogenic bladder following spinal cord injury. In: Kirshblum S, Campagnolo DI, DeLisa JA, eds. *Spinal Cord Medicine.* Philadelphia: Lippincott Williams & Wilkins; 2002:181–206.

Bowel Management: Antegrade Continence Enema

Jonathan M. Vapnek MD

Description
The antegrade continence enema allows people with significant fecal incontinence uncontrolled with a bowel routine to achieve bowel continence without the need for permanent diversion (colostomy) and without the need for an external appliance.

Key Principles
- The antegrade continence enema was first described in 1990 by Malone.
- Antegrade colonic washout produces complete colonic emptying.
- Continent catheterizable stoma allows access to the colon through the abdominal wall using a standard rubber or plastic catheter.
- The appendix is generally used as the catheterizable channel and, as originally described, was reimplanted into the cecum in a nonrefluxing fashion (the Mitrofanoff principle).
- More recent surgical modifications involve using the appendix in situ and using a laparoscopic technique.

Indications
- People with refractory fecal incontinence or constipation who have not responded to more conservative measures
- People and/or caregivers who have adequate hand function to allow insertion of a catheter into an abdominal stoma

Contraindications
- People and/or caregivers without adequate manual dexterity to perform catheterization of an abdominal stoma
- People who have responded to more conservative measures for treatment of fecal incontinence
- People who are not candidates for surgery performed under general anesthesia
- People without an appendix who cannot spare any further loss of bowel length

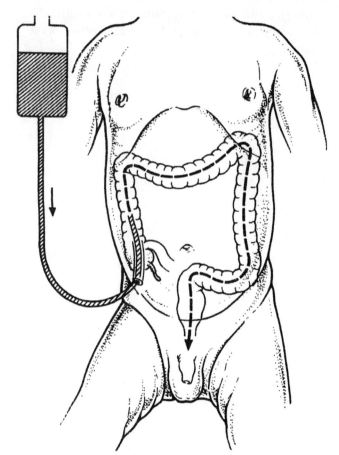

Antegrade continence enema (Reprinted with permission from Malone PSJ. Malone procedure for antegrade continence enemas. In: Spitz L, Coran AG, eds. *Rob and Smith's Operative Surgery: Pediatric Surgery*. 5th ed. London: Chapman & Hall Medical; 1995:459–467).

Special Considerations
- In those people without an appendix, a segment of intestine can be used to create the catheterizable channel.
- Even people with poor anal sphincter function are candidates, as long as the entire colon can be emptied during the washout.
- There is no consensus regarding the ideal solution to be used for the washout—neither the type nor the volume of solution has been standardized.

Key Procedural Steps

- Preoperative bowel preparation
- Prophylactic antibiotics
- Open abdominal incision or laparoscopic approach based upon surgeon preference
- Mobilization of the cecum and appendix
- Testing the appendix to confirm an adequate lumen for catheterization and length to reach the umbilicus or right lower quadrant
- Either reimplantation of appendix into the cecum or reinforcement of in situ appendix
- Creation of abdominal stoma in umbilicus or right lower quadrant

Anticipated Problems

- If appendix absent or inadequate, a catheterizable channel can be created using plicated bowel.
- Stomal stenosis is the most common complication; it can be avoided by meticulous surgical technique and use of a skin flap into the stoma.
- Stomal stenosis can be treated with dilation, surgical revision, or placement of a gastrostomy button.
- Stomal leakage is very rare but may require revision if it does occur.

Helpful Hints

- Without proven superiority of any particular surgical technique, the choice of operative approach and technique should be made by the surgeon based on his/her experience.
- Surgeons need to be flexible when performing these procedures and be able to modify their technique based on intraoperative findings.
- People and caregivers need to be carefully evaluated preoperatively to make sure that they are good candidates for the procedure.

Suggested Readings

Hensle TW, Reiley EA, Chang DT. The Malone antegrade continence enema procedure in the management of patients with spina bifida. *J Am Coll Surg.* 1998;186:669–674.

Herndon CDA, Rink RC, Cain MP, et al. In situ Malone antegrade continence enema in 127 patients: a 6-year experience. *J Urol.* 2004;172:1689–1691.

Karpman E, Das S, Kurzrock EA. Laparoscopic antegrade continence enema (Malone) procedure: description and illustration of technique. *J Endourol.* 2002;16:325–328.

Lynch AC, Beasley SW, Robertson RW, Morreau PN. Comparison of results of laparoscopic and open antegrade continence enema procedures. *Pediatr Surg Int.* 1999;15:343–346.

Malone PS, Ransley PG, Kiely EM. Preliminary report: the antegrade continence enema. *Lancet.* 1990;336:1217–1218.

Cardiovascular Exercise

Kristjan T. Ragnarsson MD

Description

Any aerobic exercise of sufficient intensity, duration, and frequency to produce increased metabolic and cardiorespiratory responses. It should be sustained for 30 to 60 minutes each time and performed 3 to 5 days each week. Intense exercise for shorter time periods also may be beneficial if repeated multiple times during the day.

Key Principles

- Persons with SCI are at increased risk for developing CVD.
- Regular aerobic exercise prevents or reduces progression of CVD, its risk factors, and comorbidities.
- Cardiovascular health benefits of aerobic exercise require sustained use of a large muscle mass.
- Aerobic exercise is muscle group specific.
- Persons with neurologically complete SCI cannot voluntarily use their largest muscle mass, that is, the lower limb muscles.
- Health benefits of upper limb aerobic exercise are significantly less than those of lower limb exercise.
- Aerobic upper limb exercise is useful and may increase aerobic capacity by 20% to 30% or more.
- The more rigorous the exercise, the greater the increases in aerobic capacity.
- Persons with SCI above T6 level have impaired cardiovascular responses to aerobic exercise due to lack of supraspinal sympathetic control.
- Training effects of aerobic exercise are lost within several weeks of exercise cessation.
- The optimal aerobic exercise intervention for persons with SCI has not been determined.
- Aerobic training effects after SCI include increased VO_2 max, cardiac output, stroke volume, decreased peripheral resistance, increased HDL and reduced LDL cholesterol, and improved glucose tolerance with increased insulin sensitivity and decreased insulin resistance.
- Lower limb muscles paralyzed by UMN lesion can be activated for aerobic exercise by functional electrical stimulation (FES) and body weight supported ambulation (BWSA).
- Aerobic exercise modalities for persons with SCI include
  - Upper limb ergometry
  - Upper limb resistance training
  - Lower limb FES ergometry
  - Hybrid exercise with simultaneous upper limb ergometry and lower limb FES ergometry
  - BWSA
  - Wheelchair sports, for example, basketball, tennis, swimming, snow skiing, track racing, and so on
  - Leisure, household, and occupational activities
  - Ambulation with gait aides and lower limb orthoses for persons with complete lower limb paralysis
  - Ambulation exercises for persons with ASIA Level D SCI.

Indications

- Increase cardiovascular fitness
- Improve carbohydrate metabolism and lipid profiles
- Prevent CVD and its comorbidities
- Increase physical and psychological well-being
- Increase bone mass

Contraindications

- Physical illness, including severe cardiopulmonary disease, for example, dysrhythmia, congestive heart failure, pulmonary disease, and so on
- Severe neuromusculoskeletal conditions affecting the limbs to be exercised

Special Considerations

- For maximum benefits, aerobic exercise should start early after SCI and gradually increase in intensity and duration.
- For sustained benefits, aerobic exercise must be done 3 to 4 times per week for 20 to 45 minutes and continued lifelong.
- Positive relationship exists between level of physical activity and quality of life in adults with SCI.
- Hybrid exercise is more effective than either upper limb or lower limb ergometry alone.
- Intense multimodal exercise can improve ASIA motor scores in chronic SCI.
- Regular aerobic exercise may reduce spasticity.
- Psychosocial benefits of regular aerobic exercise may be considerable.

Key Procedural Steps

- Set specific and realistic goals

■ Select the optimal form of aerobic exercise for each individual based on the person's physical and neurologic condition, personal interests, available training opportunities, and cost

Anticipated Problems

■ Lack of facilities providing desirable aerobic exercise training opportunities
■ Exercise-related injuries
■ Upper extremity overuse
■ Poor compliance
■ Insufficient insurance benefits

Suggested Readings

Slater D, Meade M. Participation in sports and recreation for persons with spinal cord injury: review and recommendations. *Neurorehabilitation*. 2007;19(2):121–129.

Warburton DER, Ang JJ, Krassioukov A, Sproule S. Cardiovascular health and exercise rehabilitation in spinal cord injury. *Top Spinal Cord Injury Rehabil*. 2007;13(1):98–122.

Communicating While Using a Ventilator

Dana Spivack David MS CCC-SLP

Description
Patients on mechanical ventilation may communicate verbally by cuff deflation alone or in concert with the use of a tracheostomy speaking valve.

Key Principles
- At least partial tracheostomy tube cuff deflation must be tolerated for verbal communication on a ventilator to occur.
- Cuff deflation allows for the air to pass through the upper airway and vibrate the vocal folds, resulting in phonation/vocalization or leak speech.
- The patient must learn how to coordinate the ventilator cycle with phonation when the cuff is simply deflated.
- Use of a one-way in-line speaking valve allows air from the ventilator into the tracheostomy tube but not back into the ventilator, forcing it to exit the airway through the vocal folds.
- Use of a one-way in-line speaking valve allows the patient to speak on both the inhalation and exhalation cycles of ventilation.

Indications
- Allows verbal communication for persons dependent on a ventilator for respiration.

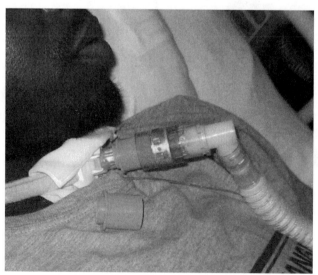

In-line speaking valve.

- Safe swallowing can be enhanced by wearing the speaking valve.
- Coughing ability can be improved by wearing the speaking valve.
- Weaning from the ventilator can be assisted by wearing the speaking valve.

Contraindications
- If the person cannot tolerate full cuff deflation, then the speaking valve cannot be placed
- Tracheal stenosis
- Vocal fold paralysis in the adduction (closed) position
- Copious amounts of secretions that need constant suctioning may limit the individual's tolerance of the speaking valve
- Severe anxiety
- Person is not awake and alert

Special Considerations
- Anxiety is very common with people on a ventilator and needs to be addressed.
- Explanations of cuff deflation and speaking valve placement should be reviewed.
- If an individual cannot achieve voice after several attempts with a speaking valve, consider referral to ENT to rule out tracheal stenosis.

Key Procedural Steps
- Educate the individual by describing how the cuff will be deflated and the speaking valve placed
- Deflate the cuff fully and allow the individual to adjust to the airflow in the upper airway
- Suction the individual prior to valve placement
- Adjust the ventilator settings by increasing the inhaled tidal volume to compensate for the air leak created by the cuff deflation
- Fit the in-line speaking valve (ie, Passy Muir Speaking Valve) in line with the ventilator tubing at the hub of the tracheostomy tube
- Instruct the individual to verbalize through a variety of speech tasks (ie, counting to 10)
- Monitor the individual's oxygen level and heart rate with a pulse oximeter

- If the individual does not tolerate the speaking valve (as evidenced by the patient's oxygen level dropping below 90%) then remove the valve
- If the individual tolerates the speaking valve, the goal is to gradually increase the amount of time that the patient wears the valve
- When the speaking valve trial is completed, remove the valve and replace the ventilator tubing
- Readjust the ventilator settings and inflate the cuff as required

Anticipated Problems
- The individual may feel too much airflow or difficulty breathing
- The tidal volume must be increased adequately to adjust for the leak that is caused by the cuff being fully deflated or the individual will not be properly ventilated

- Ventilator alarms need to be adjusted to avoid their sounding due to the air leaks
- Coughing while adjusting to the airflow to the nose and mouth
- Anxiety

Helpful Hints
- Explain the procedure to the patient prior to the speaking valve placement in order to lessen anxiety
- Suction the patient prior to speaking valve placement, as copious secretions can reduce tolerance of the valve

Suggested Reading
Dikeman Karen J, Kazandjian Marta S. *Communication and Swallowing Management of Tracheostomized and Ventilator-Dependent Adults.* 2nd ed. New York: Thomson Delmar Learning; 2003.

Section II: Interventions

Health Maintenance

Avniel Shetreat-Klein MD PhD

Description
Advances in surgical and rehabilitative care have dramatically lengthened life spans in patients with SCI. As a result, mortality in patients with SCI is increasingly due to the same chronic health conditions that affect the population at large. Therefore, preventative care and reduction of modifiable risk factors play an important role in maintaining the health of patients with SCI.

Key Principles
- Some health maintenance principles are specific to persons with SCI, and are directly related to an individual's impairments (eg, respiratory care, bladder management, skin care).
- Other health maintenance principles apply to all adults (eg, minimizing cardiovascular risk factors, cancer screenings).

Indications
- All people require regular attention to health maintenance.

Special Considerations
- Referral to a primary care specialist is indicated to ensure that general health maintenance guidelines are followed.

Key Procedural Steps

Skin
- Daily examination of skin is required for anyone with impaired sensation or mobility due to the risk of pressure ulcers.
- Skin should be checked for new or changed pigmented lesions.
- Suspicious lesions should be biopsied. Basal cell carcinomas can be mistaken for nonhealing wounds.

Respiratory
- Individuals with impaired thoracic musculature are at risk for respiratory infections due to poor clearing of secretions and hypoaeration.
- Individuals and caregivers should be instructed in pulmonary toilet and assisted cough.
- Yearly influenza vaccines and pneumonia vaccines every 5 years are recommended.
- Counseling and treatment for smoking cessation is imperative.

Cardiovascular
- Individuals with SCI are at higher risk for cardiovascular complications than the general population.
- Special attention therefore should be paid to regular blood pressure and lipid screening.
- Address modifiable risk factors.

Metabolic/Endocrine
- Obesity occurs at a higher rate in the SCI population.
- Weighing people in wheelchairs can be a challenge, but obesity carries with it a significant burden of additional morbidity and should be monitored and addressed promptly.
- Glucose intolerance and diabetes occur at a higher rate in the SCI population and the American Diabetes Association recommendations suggest screening every 3 years or less.
- Osteoporosis occurs at a higher rate in the SCI population.
- Individuals should start calcium and vitamin D treatment soon after injury and bisphosphonate use should be considered in the nonambulatory.

Gastrointestinal
- Constipation and diarrhea should be prevented with use of an appropriate bowel routine.
- Ulcer prevention with a proton-pump inhibitor is typically initiated soon after SCI and continued for 3 months.
- Individuals with SCI are at higher lifetime risk for gastrointestinal bleeding, and may be less sensitive to the painful symptoms that call attention to potential ulcers.
- Screening for colorectal cancer begins at age 50 for both men and women.
- Use of a lidocaine anal block may prevent autonomic dyreflexia associated with colonoscopy.

Reproductive/urinary
- Individuals with neurogenic bladder should have yearly screening with renal and bladder ultrasound to rule out hydronephrosis and stones.
- Creatinine levels should be monitored as an assessment of kidney function.

- Persistent hematuria, especially in the setting of an indwelling catheter, should trigger referral to a urologist for cystoscopy to rule out carcinoma.
- Annual prostate-specific antigen (PSA) testing and digital rectal exam should be performed annually in males above the age of 50 (45 in high-risk populations).
- In females, breast cancer screening begins as early as age 18 in high-risk populations.
- The recommended interval for cervical cancer screening is 1 year.

Musculoskeletal
- Teach and reinforce proper mobility techniques to avoid repetitive stress injuries

Equipment
- Routinely check individuals' wheelchair(s) and ask about the state of their adaptive equipment, assistive devices, or orthotics

- Improperly maintained, damaged, or poorly fitting equipment puts patients at risk for injury

Helpful Hints
- Health maintenance/preventative care issues should be addressed on every visit, whether directly or by ensuring appropriate primary care follow-up.
- Making this a regular component of office visit will help to minimize preventable health problems.

Suggested Readings
Klingbeil H, Baer HR, Wilson PE. Aging with a disability. *Arch Phys Med Rehabil.* 2004;85:68–73.

U.S. Department of Health and Human Services, Agency of Healthcare Research and Quality. *The Guide to Clinical Preventive Services, Recommendations of the U.S. Preventive Services Task Force.* 2007.

Section II: Interventions

Home Modifications

Kristjan T. Ragnarsson MD

Description

Home modification is the remodeling of an existing or new home to make it accessible to a specific physically impaired individual or to all people, regardless of their physical mobility skills (universal design).

Key Principles

- Start with home evaluation by reviewing floor plans
- Make a home visit
- Recommend architectural changes
- Contract with an architect and a builder
- Focus on general features, entrances, bathrooms, kitchens, bedrooms, stairs, and laundry area

Indications

- Mobility impairment that requires wheelchair and/or assistive gait devices
- Risk of falling

Contraindications

- None, preferably all homes, should be accessible to all persons, regardless of their mobility status.

Special Considerations

General features

- A single floor dwelling is optimal, but at least the bedroom, bathroom, and kitchen should be on the same floor
- Doorways: 32 to 36 inches wide
- Hallways: >36 inches wide
- Light switches: 36 to 42 inches from floor
- Electrical outlets: >15 inches from floor
- Window sills: <30 inches from floor
- Thermostats: 36 inches from floor
- Adequate, even lighting in all areas
- Doors should have lever-style handles (not knobs)
- Level or beveled thresholds <1/2 inch in height
- Doors with offset hinges to maximize width of open doorways

Entrances

- Ramp incline: preferably 1:20 or at least 1:12

- Long ramps are divided into 10- to 12-foot sections with platforms between
- Nonslip ramp surface with fire-resistant construction
- A space 5 feet by 5 for door management at ramp's top and bottom and at any ramp turns
- Easy-to-reach door locks

Bathrooms

- Should be located adjacent to or near the bedroom
- Size: more than 8 feet by 10 feet
- Sinks with open space underneath for knee clearance
- Sink pipes behind walls or well recessed
- Faucet handles are of lever type
- Standard height toilet, if commode-chair is used
- Tub/shower seat, built-in or set-in
- Roll-in shower: more than 5 feet by 5 feet, nonslip floor, sloped for water drainage
- Handheld shower head with 6-foot hose and built-in on/off control
- Thermostat set for <120° water temperature
- Mirrors and cabinets are set low
- Strategically placed grab bars

Kitchen

- Countertops: 30 to 35 inches above floor with 24-inch space underneath for knee clearance
- Cabinet doors and drawers easy to open/close and placed at proper heights
- Stove height 30 to 32 inches with large front-mounted control knobs
- Ovens set low at individual discretion
- Side by side refrigerator/freezer with self-defrosting

Bedroom

- Minimum size: 10 feet by 14 feet with 5- by 5-foot clear area and a 3-foot-wide passage to bed and bathroom
- Closets with accessible shelves less than 4 feet 6 inches from floor and rods for hanging clothes less than 4 feet from floor
- Telephone and light switch should be easily reachable from bed

Stairs

- Sturdy handrails extending beyond the top and bottom of stairs

- Light switches placed at top and bottom of stairs
- Step height: 6 to 7 inches with depth >10 inches

Laundry

- Preferably located on main floor
- Front-loading washers and dryers
- Table for folding clothes 30 to 32 inches in height

Key Procedural Steps

- Plan well in a timely manner
- Obtain estimates from three contractors
- Secure financing for construction

Anticipated Problems

- Inadequate design
- Inadequate construction

Helpful Hints

- Have the person with SCI and their family visit properly renovated homes

Suggested Reading

Hsiao I, Hodne T. Architectural considerations for improving access. In: Lin VW, ed. *Spinal Cord Medicine Principles and Practice*. New York: Demos; 2003:975–986.

Inferior Vena Cava Filters

Greg Nemunaitis MD

Description
An inferior vena cava (IVC) filter is a medical device that is implanted into the IVC to prevent pulmonary emboli (PE).

Key Principles
- PE is the third leading cause of death in the first year following SCI.
- The incidence of PE in individuals with acute SCI is 2.6%.
- Filters significantly decrease the risk of PE.
- Filters will decrease the risk of PE but increase the risk of deep vein thrombosis (DVT).
- Filters do not prevent PE related to upper extremity DVT.
- Filters are available that are retrievable.
  - Retrievable filters are made with an attachment such as a small hook or loop that allows them to be snared and pulled back into a sheath and removed through the jugular vein.
- Filters can be placed through the femoral vein, the internal jugular vein, or an arm vein with one design.
- Filters are typically placed just below the lowest renal vein.
- Filters are placed above the renal veins in pregnant patients or women of childbearing age or those with renal venous thromboembolism (VTE).
- Consider filter removal at 8 weeks post-SCI in individuals with incomplete motor injuries who do not have VTE or additional risk factors for VTE, eg, lower limb fractures, a history of thrombosis, cancer, heart failure, obesity, or age over 70.
- Consider filter removal at 12 weeks post-SCI in individuals who do not have VTE and who have complete motor injuries or incomplete motor injuries with additional risk factors for VTE, eg, lower limb fractures, a history of thrombosis, cancer, heart failure, obesity, or age over 70.

Indications
- Failed anticoagulant prophylaxis with development of DVT or PE despite adequate anticoagulation
- Contraindication to anticoagulation
- Complication of anticoagulation such as hemorrhage or thrombocytopenia

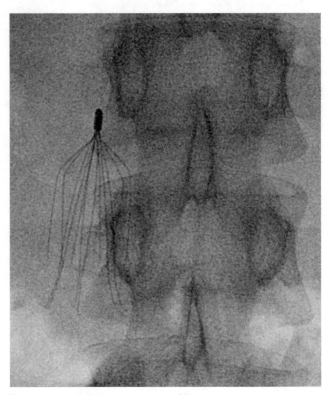

Removable inferior vena cava filter.

- Large VTE within the IVC or iliac veins
- Consider in persons with complete motor SCI due to lesions in the high cervical cord (C2, C3) and in those with poor cardiopulmonary reserve

Contraindications
- Uncorrectable, severe coagulopathy
- Bacteremia
- Extensive IVC thrombosis such that placement of a filter between the VTE and pulmonary circulation is not possible

Special Considerations
- Successful retrieval of filter is more difficult the longer the filter has been in place.
- Ultrasound-guided venous micropuncture enables filter placement to be performed without full reversal of anticoagulation as the risk of arterial puncture is minimized.

Procedural Steps

- Choose a retrievable IVC filter design
- Choose a femoral or internal jugular route of placement depending on the amount and location of VTE
- Insert catheter into the IVC under fluoroscopic guidance
- Perform a venogram of the IVC to assess for potential anatomic variations, thrombi within the IVC, and areas of stenoses
- Advance the catheter to the desired location below the lowest renal vein
- Advance the filter through the catheter and deploy just below the lowest renal vein
- Obtain a postinsertion X-ray to assess filter position

Anticipated Problems

- Filter malposition
- DVT at the needle puncture site
- Filter migration
- Vena cava thrombosis
- Renal vein thrombosis
- Filter thrombosis
- Fractured filter strut
- Recurrent pulmonary embolism with the filter in place is reported in 2% to 5% of patients

Helpful Hints

- Remove filter as soon as it is appropriate

Suggested Readings

Becker DM, Philbrick JT, Selby JB. Inferior vena caval filters. Indications, safety, effectiveness. *Arch Intern Med.* 1992;152:1985–1994.

Decousus H, Leizorovicz A, Parent F, et al. A clinical trial of vena caval filters in the prevention of pulmonary embolism in patients with proximal deep vein thrombosis. *N Engl J Med.* 1998;338:409–415.

Johns J, Nguyen C, Sing RF. Vena cava filters in spinal cord injuries: evolving technology. *Spinal Cord Med.* 2006;29(3):183–190.

Rogers FB, Shackford S, Ricci M, Wilson J, Parsons S. Routine prophylactic vena caval filter insertion in severely injured trauma patients decreases the incidence of pulmonary embolism. *J Am Coll Surg.* 1995;180:641–647.

Intrathecal Pump: Evaluation and Placement

Thomas N. Bryce MD

Description
An intrathecal (IT) medication pump is an implantable device that can allow continuous and/or bolus dosing of medication directly into the intrathecal space.

Key Principles
- Medications can be administered intrathecally to increase the concentration of the drug at the target receptors within the spinal cord without the sedating effects of systemically administered oral medications.
- Baclofen is the most commonly used IT drug for treating spasticity.
- Morphine is the most commonly used IT drug for treating pain.
- Zoconotoxin, a neurotoxin derived from the sea snail, is also FDA approved in the United States for IT use for treating pain.

Indications

Spasticity
- Spasticity, which causes significant pain, interferes with function, or interferes with hygiene and is uncontrolled by stretching, maximally tolerated doses of oral medications, or local treatments

Pain
- Chronic pain, which causes significant distress or interferes with function and is uncontrolled by maximally tolerated doses of oral medications, psychologic treatments, or local treatments

Contraindications
- Unable, unwilling, or thought to be unreliable by healthcare provider to follow up regularly for IT pump refills
- Presence of active infection
- Allergy to the medications, which would be infused into the pump
- Unsuccessful test dose of intrathecal medication
- Severe spinal stenosis, which would preclude placement of catheter tubing within canal adjacent the neural elements
- Pump cannot be implanted 2.5 cm or less from the skin surface

Special Considerations
- As the lumbar-cervical baclofen concentration gradient is 4:1, it should be noted that the effect will be greater in the legs rather than the arms.
- If a person has troublesome upper extremity spasticity, the pump catheter tip should be advanced and located within the upper thoracic spine.
- If a person has only troublesome lower extremity spasticity, the pump catheter tip should located within the lower thoracic spine.
- If a person has only nonspasm-related pain, the pump catheter tip should located within the lumbar spine in order to minimize neural compromise if a catheter tip granuloma should develop.

Key Procedural Steps

Intrathecal screening test trial
- Educate regarding screening test procedure and obtain written informed consent.
- If drug to be used is baclofen, perform lumbar puncture to intrathecally administer 50 to 100 mcg of preservative-free baclofen.
- If drug to be used is morphine, perform lumbar puncture to intrathecally administer 0.2 to 1 mg of preservative-free morphine.
- Keep supine for 3 hours
- Allow test subject to get up and perform usual activities, especially those activities which provoke spasticity or pain while monitoring the subjective and objective response.

Pump implantation
- Mark pump pocket site while patient is sitting
- Place distal spinal catheter within the IT space using a paramedian oblique approach
- Prepare the pump pocket in the lower abdomen away from the iliac crest and the belt line
- Tunnel the proximal pump catheter in the subcutaneous tissue from the spinal incision to the pump pocket
- Trim distal catheter segment to desired length

- Connect proximal and distal catheters segments in the back and anchor to the fascia
- Connect proximal catheter to pump, place pump in pocket, and suture pump to the fascia

Anticipated Problems
- Baclofen overdose can manifest with respiratory depression and hypotension, and these vital signs should be closely monitored.
- Morphine overdose can manifest with respiratory depression, central nervous system depression, seizures, and respiratory arrest.
- Have the narcotic antagonist, naloxone, available during opioid screening trial.

Helpful Hints
- If patient is nonambulatory, consider using 100 mcg baclofen to ensure adequate response for trial.

- If ambulatory, consider using 50 mcg baclofen to avoid excessive weakness.
- Calculate the intrathecal morphine daily dose equivalent and administer this dose for the trial for persons on chronic oral opioids; for oral morphine, the oral to intrathecal dose conversion is 300:1.
- Do not hold all of the standing opioids the day of the trial unless they have been tapered in the weeks preceding the trial in order to avoid opioid withdrawal; but, consider giving half of the oral opioid dosage for the day of the trial to avoid oversedation.
- The initial effect should be seen 3 to 4 hours after trial injection and should wear off within 24 hours.

Suggested Reading
Medtronic Syncromed II Clinical Reference Guide. Minneapolis: Medtronic Neurological; 2004.

Intrathecal Pump: Management

Thomas N. Bryce MD

Description

An intrathecal (IT) medication pump is an implantable device, which can allow continuous and/or bolus dosing of medication directly into the intrathecal space.

Key Principles

- Medications should be started at low doses and titrated to the lowest effective dose.
- Scheduled refills with reprogramming range from <1 month to 6 months depending on the concentration of medication and its rate of administration.
- Scheduled replacements of the implanted pump based upon expected battery life range from 5 to 7 years.
- Deaths have been reported when pump refills have been missed.

Indications

- Finding a therapeutic dose
- Maintaining therapy effectiveness
- Evaluating a loss of effectiveness
- Identifying and preventing complications

Special Considerations

- Both a reliable and vigilant patient or caregiver as well as a responsive pump management team is essential for avoiding the potentially devastating complications of medication withdrawal.

Key Procedural Steps

Finding the appropriate dose

- Start with 50 to 100 mcg/day simple continuous dosing for baclofen.
- Start with daily oral equivalent dose of morphine.
- Increase the rate every 3 days or more by 10% to 30% until an effective dose is obtained.
- Reduce the oral medications that IT medications are replacing slowly over several weeks after implantation.

Refill procedure

- Interrogate pump with programmer to confirm need for refill, size of reservoir, type and concentration of medication(s).
- Acquire needed supplies and prepare medications.
- Prepare skin over pump.
- Place template over pump reservoir and access using noncoring needle.

- Remove old medication noting amount and comparing to what is expected to be removed.
- Refill reservoir with new medication.
- Reinterrogate and reprogram pump with the amount of medication infused, its concentration, current rate, and volume at which alarm will be triggered.
- Recheck programming.

Addressing a mild loss of effect of IT medication

- Interrogate pump to confirm there is medication in reservoir.
- Ensure that refill is not imminently or past due as these could result in a lower rate of medication administration.
- Look for local or systemic causes of increased pain or spasticity such as infection or pressure ulcers.
- If side effects are not present or tolerable, increase intrathecal dose of medication.

Addressing a severe loss of effect of IT medication

- Interrogate pump to confirm there is medication in reservoir.
- Access pump to check to see that amount of medication within reservoir is as expected.
- Give test bolus through pump reprogramming and observe for effect.
- For suspected pump failure not at the end of the life expectance of the batteries, a rotor study can be performed whereby a specific rapid bolus can be administered under fluoroscopic observation of the pump rotor.
- For a suspected catheter problem, image pump and spine to look for any obvious disconnections and to see if catheter is within canal.
- If no incongruities have been found, infuse contrast through the side access port of the pump under fluoroscopy to confirm catheter placement.
- Infusion of radiolabeled material into the pump reservoir is an alternate method of confirming the catheter placement.

Anticipated Problems

Problems that require surgical intervention

- Spinal epidural hematoma (early complication)

- Catheter kinking, disconnection, leakage, breakage, or occlusion
- Catheter migration out of intrathecal space
- Catheter tip fibrosis and inflammatory granuloma formation
- Pump or telemetry component failure
- Loss of battery charge
- Erosion of pump out of pocket through skin
- Pump pocket infection

Problems that typically do not require surgical intervention

- Medication overdose
- Medication withdrawal
- Spinal headache due to cerebral spinal fluid leak
- Pump pocket seroma or hematoma
- Spinal hygroma at site of lumbar incision

- Arachnoiditis
- Meningitis

Helpful Hints

- Always use preservative-free medication to avoid arachnoiditis.
- Be aware of the risk of medication precipitating out of solution if used at higher than standard concentrations and in untested combinations.
- Specific programmed boluses of medication can be useful for times when pain or spasticity is most troublesome.
- Patient-controlled modules are available for use when increases of pain are unpredictable.

Suggested Reading

Medtronic. *Medtronic Syncromed II Clinical Reference Guide.* Minneapolis: Medtronic Neurological; 2004.

Limb Orthoses

Donald Macron MD MA ■ Richard Freiden MD

Description
Limb orthoses are external devices that protect limb anatomy, correct misalignment, prevent contracture, or maximize function by assisting with position and mobility.

Key Principles
- Appropriate device selection depends primarily upon motor level and severity of SCI.
- Sensory level is important for feedback and comfort.
- The prescriber specifies which joints are crossed and how they are affected (ie, assist or resist movement, provide support, etc.).
- Goal-setting guides device selection, considering the individual's capabilities, needs, and desires.
- Devices are prefabricated and custom-fitted, or custom-made to specific measurements.
- Bracing nomenclature is based on abbreviations, using the first letter of each joint crossed—proximal to distal—followed by the distal region of attachment (eg, an HKAFO is a hip-knee-ankle-foot orthosis).

Indications
- To maintain functional limb position and joint ROM
- To stabilize weakened limbs and protect insensate areas from injury
- To improve comfort and hygiene

Contraindications
- Avoid use in cases where orthoses cannot ensure sufficient stability, protection, or immobilization to a compromised region.
- Avoid contact with open wounds or pressure to insensate, vulnerable soft tissues.
- Use with caution on body parts with fluctuating size and shape (eg, edema, weight change, dialysis, etc.).

Special Considerations
- Orthosis selection is influenced by device weight and size, cosmesis, comfort, ease of use, durability, and cost effectiveness.
- Individuals and caregivers need instruction on the device's purpose, routine care, correct positioning and fit, monitoring for pressure points and irritation, and identifying device malfunction.
- A functional assessment performed 1 month postinjury helps delineate long-term vs. short-term impairments and goals.

Key Procedural Steps
- Fit and alignment should be checked prior to orthosis customization, and after using a new device for at least 20 minutes.
- Evaluate for impingement and brace migration

Anticipated Problems
- Atrophy or weakness may occur in immobilized areas.
- Skin breakdown may occur when worn on an insensate limb.
- Spasticity is a limiting factor in the use of orthoses.
- Incorrectly applied devices can disrupt the standing balance or gait of an otherwise functional individual.
- Due to their solid design and rigid materials, some devices can be hot and retain moisture.

Helpful Hints
- Braces and functional electrical stimulation are often used concurrently, although more for health benefits than for mobility.
- Are standing and walking viable goals? KAFOs or Vannini-Rizzoli AFOs and crutches can allow ambulation by persons who have a neurological level between T11 and L2.
- AFOs can allow ambulation by persons who have a neurological level at or below L3.
- Increased energy expenditure during ambulation occurs with increased severity of SCI.
- Prescriptions should include joint type and locking mechanism.
- Reciprocating gait orthoses are variants of bilateral HKAFOs that may help persons with high paraplegia ambulate short distances with high-energy expenditure for exercise.
- Individuals with a C5 motor level can use universal cuffs (adapters to hold utensils, pencils, etc),

long opponens splints, and ratchet wrist hand orthoses (WHO). The balanced forearm orthosis assists hand placement when shoulder and elbow muscles are weak.

- Individuals with weak wrist extensors should be prescribed splints that support the wrist in order to prevent stretching of the wrist and finger extensor tendons, which are necessary for tenodesis.
- Individuals with a C6 motor level can use cuffs- or wrist-driven WHO (which create dynamic finger prehension through wrist extension).

- Individuals with a C8 motor level can use a static hand orthosis with a lumbrical bar and thumb post to prevent "clawing."

Suggested Readings

Garber SL, Gregorio TL. Upper extremity assistive devices: assessment of use by spinal cord-injured patients with quadriplegia. *Am J Occup Ther.* 1990;44(2):126–131.

Jaeger RJ, Yarkony GM, Roth EJ. Rehabilitation technology for standing and walking after spinal cord injury. *Am J Phys Med Rehabil.* 1989;68(3):128–133.

Loke M. New concepts in lower limb orthotics. *Phys Med Rehab Clin NA.* 2000;11:477–496.

Neurologic Classification of Spinal Cord Injury

Adam B. Stein MD

Description
Once the examiner has performed a complete sensory, motor, and anorectal examination, the sensory levels, motor levels, single neurologic level, completeness of injury, ASIA Impairment Scale (AIS) and, if pertinent, zone of partial preservation (ZPP) are determined.

Key Principles
- The sensory level is the most caudal dermatome where both light touch and pinprick are normal.
- A different sensory level may be determined for the right and the left side of the body.
- The motor level is the most caudal muscle having grade 3 or better strength where all muscles above are graded 5.
- A different motor level may be determined for the right and left side of the body.
- The single neurologic level is the most rostral of the sensory and motor levels.
- A complete injury is defined as the absence of both sensory and motor functions in S4-S5.
- An incomplete injury is defined as the presence of sensory or motor function in S4-S5.
- The ZPP is used only for complete injuries.
- The ZPP is the most caudal level that has sensory and/or motor function below the level of injury. There may be four distinct recordings for the ZPP (sensory, motor, left , right).
- The AIS is a five-point scale used to specify the severity of the injury.
  - AIS "A" is a complete injury.
  - AIS "B" has sensory, but no motor function present more than three levels below the neurologic level, and includes S4-S5.
  - AIS "C" has motor function present more than three levels below the neurologic level but the majority of key muscles below the level are less than grade 3, and sensory or motor function at S4-S5 is present.
  - AIS "D" has motor function present more than three levels below the neurologic level, at least half the key muscles below the level are grade 3 or better, and sensory or motor function at S4-S5 is present.
  - AIS "E": All components of the standardized exam are normal.

Key Procedural Steps
- Determine the sensory level for each side of the body.
- Determine the motor level for each side of the body.
- Determine the single neurologic level defined as the most rostral of the four sensory/motor levels.
- Determine whether injury is complete or incomplete by referring to the results of the anorectal exam.
- Determine the AIS grade.
- If the injury is AIS level A, determine the ZPP.

Anticipated Problems
- If the level of injury is at a site for which there is no key muscle (eg, C2-C4, T2-L1, S2-S4/S5), the motor level is defined by the sensory level.
- If exactly 50% of the muscles below the level of injury are grade 3 or better, the correct AIS classification is D.
- If an individual has motor function more than three levels below the neurological level and sensory or motor function at S4-S5 is present, the injury is motor incomplete, even if the only muscle to demonstrate such activity is not a key muscle.
- Reflex function observed during rectal exam has no bearing on determination of completeness or AIS grade.

Helpful Hints
- Volitional contraction of the rectal sphincter is evidence of a motor incomplete injury, even if there is no voluntary movement of a limb muscle below the level of injury.
- If it is clear that a sensory or motor deficit is not a result of the SCI, those dermatomes and myotomes so affected are considered normal for the purpose of classification.

Suggested Readings

American Spinal Injury Association. *Reference Manual for the International Standards for Neurological Classification of Spinal Cord Injury.* Chicago, IL: American Spinal Injury Association; 2003:46–60.

Marino RJ, Barros T, Biering-Sorensen, et al. International standards for neurological classification of spinal cord injury. *J Spinal Cord Med.* 2003;26(Suppl 1):S50–S56.

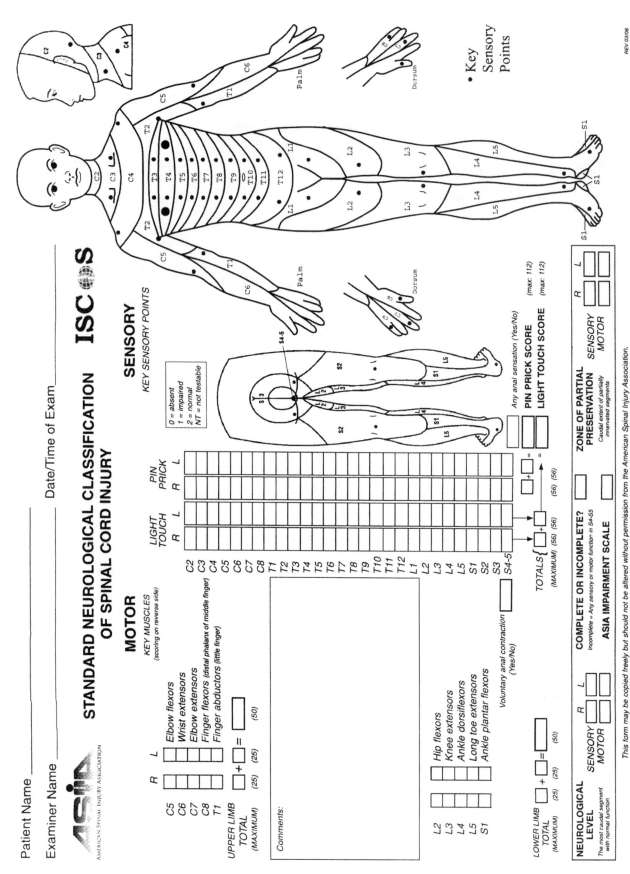

MUSCLE GRADING

0 total paralysis

1 palpable or visible contraction

2 active movement, full range of motion, gravity eliminated

3 active movement, full range of motion, against gravity

4 active movement, full range of motion, against gravity and provides some resistance

5 active movement, full range of motion, against gravity and provides normal resistance

5* muscle able to exert, in examiner's judgement, sufficient resistance to be considered normal if identifiable inhibiting factors were not present

NT not testable. Patient unable to reliably exert effort or muscle unavailable for testing due to factors such as immobilization, pain on effort or contracture.

ASIA IMPAIRMENT SCALE

☐ **A = Complete**: No motor or sensory function is preserved in the sacral segments S4-S5.

☐ **B = Incomplete**: Sensory but not motor function is preserved below the neurological level and includes the sacral segments S4-S5.

☐ **C = Incomplete**: Motor function is preserved below the neurological level, and more than half of key muscles below the neurological level have a muscle grade less than 3.

☐ **D = Incomplete**: Motor function is preserved below the neurological level, and at least half of key muscles below the neurological level have a muscle grade of 3 or more.

☐ **E = Normal**: Motor and sensory function are normal.

CLINICAL SYNDROMES (OPTIONAL)

☐ Central Cord
☐ Brown-Sequard
☐ Anterior Cord
☐ Conus Medullaris
☐ Cauda Equina

STEPS IN CLASSIFICATION

The following order is recommended in determining the classification of individuals with SCI.

1. Determine sensory levels for right and left sides.

2. Determine motor levels for right and left sides.
   Note: in regions where there is no myotome to test, the motor level is presumed to be the same as the sensory level.

3. Determine the single neurological level.
   This is the lowest segment where motor and sensory function is normal on both sides, and is the most cephalad of the sensory and motor levels determined in steps 1 and 2.

4. Determine whether the injury is Complete or Incomplete (sacral sparing).
   If voluntary anal contraction = No AND all S4-5 sensory scores = 0 AND any anal sensation = No, then injury is COMPLETE. Otherwise injury is incomplete.

5. Determine ASIA Impairment Scale (AIS) Grade:
   Is injury Complete? If YES, AIS=A Record ZPP
   (For ZPP record lowest dermatome or myotome on each side with some (non-zero score) preservation)

   NO

   Is injury motor incomplete? If NO. AIS=B
   (Yes=voluntary anal contraction OR motor function more than three levels below the motor level on a given side.)

   YES

   Are at least half of the key muscles below the (single) neurological level graded 3 or better?

   NO   YES
   AIS=C   AIS=D

If sensation and motor function is normal in all segments, AIS=E
Note: AIS E is used in follow up testing when an individual with a documented SCI has recovered normal function. If at initial testing no deficits are found, the individual is neurologically intact; the ASIA Impairment Scale does not apply.

Standard neurologic classification of spinal cord injury.

Neurologic Examination: Motor Testing

Adam B. Stein MD

Description

Motor testing is performed to determine the most caudal level of normal motor function and to identify the presence, location, and magnitude of motor function below the level of injury.

Key Principles

- Motor testing requires examination of 10 key muscles on each side of the body: 5 in the upper limb and 5 in the lower limb.
- Each key muscle represents a single myotome.
- The five upper limb key muscles represent the C5–T1 myotomes; the lower limb key muscles represent the L2–S1 myotomes.
- For myotomes not assigned a key muscle, the sensory exam is used to reflect motor function at that level.
- Each key muscle is scored 0–5 according to standard muscle testing principles.
- "+" or "−" grades are not utilized.
- A grade of 5* is utilized if the tested muscle is judged by the examiner to have normal strength but the presence of a mitigating factor, such as pain, precludes demonstration of that strength.
- A muscle scored grade 3 or better is considered normal.
- In reality, no key muscles are innervated by a single spinal segment. For the purposes of classification, a muscle scored grade 3 is considered to be normally innervated by the most rostral of its innervating spinal levels; therefore, the muscle is considered normal for that myotome.
- Motor level is defined as most caudal level with muscle strength 3 or greater if muscle one segment rostral is graded 5.
- When there is no key muscle immediately rostral to a key muscle graded 3 or 4, use the sensory exam as indicative of motor function at that more rostral level.
- A motor level is determined for each side of the body, right and left.

Indications

- The motor exam should be performed on all persons with SCI.

Contraindications

- Individual is unable to understand instructions or participate in examination

Special Considerations

- Performing the motor examination at 72 hours after injury allows the examiner to perform an accurate exam in the vast majority of cases.

Key Procedural Steps

- The motor examination is performed with the individual supine.
- Examine each muscle in the grade 3 (antigravity) position first.
- If the individual demonstrates grade 3 strength, test for grade 4 or 5.
- If the individual does not have grade 3 strength, place the muscle in the gravity eliminated position to determine if the strength is 0, 1, or 2.
- The motor exam should be performed in a rostral to caudal direction in the order of the myotomes.
- Record the muscle grade for each muscle on a standard examination sheet available from ASIA and reprinted on pages 140–141.

Anticipated Problems

- Improper positioning of the individual may lead to muscle substitution and the potential for inaccurate muscle grading.
- Be attentive to the potential for trace muscle contraction as overlooking the presence of minimal contraction may result in erroneous prognostication of outcome.
- The presence of contractures may cause confusion and inaccuracy in muscle grading.
- If 50% of the range is unavailable, the muscle cannot be accurately scored and is recorded as "not testable" (NT).
- Do not grade up; if the muscle tests as not quite a 4, the proper grade would be a 3.
- Muscle spasticity may mimic volitional motor function.
- Strength testing in the presence of pain may be unreliable.

Helpful Hints

- When a key muscle is unavailable for testing, the muscle should be scored NT and the reason why noted.
- If the individual demonstrates the ability to volitionally contract a muscle that is not one of the key muscles, this should be noted.
- In the presence of spasticity, the examiner should attempt to relax the muscle to allow for accurate grading. If this is impossible, score the muscle NT.
- If the individual has an associated condition affecting muscle strength, and the strength decrement is not related to the SCI, note this in the comment section (eg, brachial plexus injury).

- Examine the muscles in the same order every time to improve reliability.
- Having a recorder document the results can improve the efficiency of the exam.

Suggested Readings

American Spinal Injury Association. *Reference Manual for the International Standards for Neurological Classification of Spinal Cord Injury.* Chicago, IL: American Spinal Injury Association; 2003:21–45.

Marino RJ, Barros T, Biering-Sorensen, et al. International standards for neurological classification of spinal cord injury. *J Spinal Cord Med.* 2003;26(Suppl 1):S50–S56.

Neurologic Examination: Motor Testing, Lower Myotomes

Kimberly Sackheim DO ■ Thomas N. Bryce MD

Description
Motor testing assess for weakness in the L2–S1 myotomes.

Key Principles
- Muscle strength is graded on a six-point scale.
- Grade 0: no visible or palpable contraction
- Grade 1: any visible or palpable contraction
- Grade 2: full range of motion with gravity eliminated
- Grade 3: full range of motion against gravity without resistance
- Grade 4: full range of motion against resistance but not normal strength
- Grade 5: normal strength

Indications
- Perform on all individuals with SCI.

Special Considerations
- Always perform with the individual supine to ensure consistency.
- If less than half of the joint ROM is available, grade the muscle as nontestable.

Key Procedural Steps

Iliopsoas—L2
- Grades 0 and 1: Flex hip 15°. While you support the thigh, palpate the muscle distal to the anterior superior iliac spine and ask the individual to flex the thigh.
- Grade 2: Fully externally rotate and flex hip 45°. Flex knee 90°. While you support the leg, ask the individual to flex the hip.
- Grade 3: Fully extend the knee and hip. While you support the leg, ask the individual to flex the hip up to 90°.
- Grades 4 and 5: Flex hip 90°. While you brace the opposite pelvis, ask the individual to keep the hip at 90° as you apply resistance trying to extend the hip.

Quadriceps—L3
- Grades 0 and 1: Flex hip and knee 15°. While you support the knee and palpate the extensors, ask the individual to extend the knee.

- Grade 2: Fully externally rotate hip and flex knee 90°. While you support the leg, ask the individual to straighten the knee.
- Grades 3 to 5: Partially flex the knee. Place your arm under the tested knee with your hand on top of the opposing knee. Ask the individual to straighten the knee. Perform with resistance for Grades 4 and 5.

Tibialis anterior—L4
- Grades 0 and 1: Fully extend the knee and hip. While you palpate the tibialis anterior, ask the individual to dorsiflex the foot.
- Grade 2: Fully externally rotate hip and flex knee to 90°. While supporting the ankle, ask the individual to dorsiflex the foot.
- Grade 3: Slightly flex the knee. While supporting at the ankle, ask the individual to dorsiflex the foot.
- Grades 4 and 5: Flex the knee slightly and place the ankle in full dorsiflexion. Ask the individual to maintain full dorsiflexion as you apply resistance.

Extensor hallucis longus—L5
- Grades 0 and 1: Fully extend the knee and hip. While you palpate the extensors of the big toe, ask the individual to dorsiflex the great toe.
- Grade 2: Fully externally rotate hip and flex knee to 90°. While supporting the ankle, ask the individual to dorsiflex the great toe.
- Grade 3: Slightly flex the knee. While supporting at the ankle, ask the individual to dorsiflex the great toe.
- Grades 4 and 5: Place the great toe in full dorsiflexion. Ask the individual to maintain full dorsiflexion as you apply resistance against it.

Gastrocnemius, soleus—S1
- Grades 0, 1, and 2: Fully externally rotate hip and flex knee 90°. While you palpate the plantar flexors, ask the individual to plantarflex the foot.
- Grade 3: Flex hip 45°. Flex the knee and place the plantar foot on a flat surface and ask the individual to lift the heel up off the surface.
- Grades 4 and 5: Fully extend the knee and hip and fully plantarflex the ankle. Ask the individual to maintain a plantarflexed position foot down as you apply resistance in an opposite direction.

Anticipated Problems

- Contraction and relaxation of the toe flexors and/ or ankle plantar flexors can falsely appear as active movement of the toe extensors and/or ankle dorsiflexors.
- Voluntary triggering of lower extremity spasticity can falsely appear as voluntary lower extremity motor function.

Helpful Hints

- Palpate muscle belly to appreciate trace contractions that might not be visible.

Suggested Reading

American Spinal Injury Association. *Reference Manual for the International Standards for Neurological Classification of Spinal Cord Injury.* Chicago, IL: American Spinal Injury Association; 2003:21–45.

Neurologic Examination: Motor Testing, Upper Myotomes

Kimberly Sackheim DO ■ Thomas N. Bryce MD

Description
Assess for weakness in C5–T1 myotomes.

Key Principles
- Muscle strength is graded on a six-point scale.
- Grade 0: no visible or palpable contraction
- Grade 1: any visible or palpable contraction
- Grade 2: full range of motion with gravity eliminated
- Grade 3: full range of motion against gravity without resistance
- Grade 4: full range of motion against resistance but not normal strength
- Grade 5: normal strength

Indications
- Perform on all individuals with SCI.

Special Considerations
- Always perform with the individual supine to ensure consistency.
- If less than half of the joint ROM is available, grade the muscle as nontestable.

Key Procedural Steps

Biceps, brachalis—C5
- Grades 0, 1, and 2: While supporting the forearm, palpate the flexors as the individual tries flex his or her elbow.
- Grade 3: Fully extend the elbow with the hand supinated. Ask the individual to flex his or her elbow.
- Grades 4 and 5: Flex the elbow to 90° with the hand supinated. Ask the individual to flex his or her elbow while you provide resistance.

Extensor carpi radialis—C6
- Grades 0, 1, and 2: Fully flex the wrist. Support the forearm in a neutral position and palpate the extensors while the individual tries to extend the wrist.
- Grade 3: Pronate and flex the wrist. Support the wrist and ask the individual to extend the wrist.
- Grades 4 and 5: Extend wrist to 90°. Apply resistance over the second radial metacarpal head with the heel

of your hand in a direction of ulnar deviation and palmar flexion.

Triceps—C7
- Grades 0 and 1: Support the forearm with the elbow at 30° from full extension. While palpating the elbow extensors, ask the individual to straighten his or her arm.
- Grade 2: While supporting the arm, fully flex the elbow and ask the individual to straighten it in a plane parallel to the ground.
- Grade 3: Fully flex the elbow with the hand lying by the individual's ear. While you support the arm, which is now perpendicular to the plane of the body, ask the individual to straighten it.
- Grades 4 and 5: Flex the elbow 45° from full extension. Ask the individual to straighten his or her arm as you apply resistance.

Flexor digitorum profundus—C8
- Grades 0, 1, and 2: Fully extend the metacarpophalangeal (MP) and proximal interphalangeal (PIP) joints. Restrict flexion of the middle PIP joint with one hand. Palpate the flexors while the individual makes a fist.
- Grade 3: Supinate the wrist with the MP and PIP joints extended. While you stabilize at the wrist, restrict flexion of the middle PIP joint with the other hand. Ask the individual to make a fist and observe for flexion of the distal interphalangeal (DIP) joint.
- Grades 4 and 5: Supinate the wrist with the MP and PIP joints extended. While you stabilize at the wrist, restrict flexion of the middle PIP joint with the other hand. Place the DIP in full flexion and ask the individual to make a fist as you apply resistance against the middle DIP.

Abductor digiti minimi—T1
- Grades 0, 1, and 2: Fully pronate the wrist with the MP, PIP, and DIP joints fully extended. While palpating the abductor digiti minimi (ADM), ask the individual to abduct the little finger.
- Grade 3: Flex the elbow to 90°, fully internally rotate the shoulder and pronate the wrist. While supporting the hand, ask the individual to abduct the little finger.
- Grades 4 and 5: Flex the elbow to 90°, fully internally rotate the shoulder and pronate the wrist. Fully abduct

the little finger and ask the individual to maintain full abduction as you apply resistance against it.

Anticipated Problems

- Elbow extension caused by volitional supination of the forearm and gravity can be falsely interpreted as volitional triceps activity.
- Finger extension associated finger abduction can be falsely interpreted as volitional ADM activity.

Helpful Hints

- Palpate muscle belly for trace contractions that might not be visible.

Suggested Reading

American Spinal Injury Association. *Reference Manual for the International Standards for Neurological Classification of Spinal Cord Injury.* Chicago: American Spinal Injury Association; 2003:21–45.

Neurologic Examination: Rectal Examination

Adam B. Stein MD

Description

The anorectal examination is a critical component of the neurologic assessment of a patient with SCI. The rectal exam has important implications for injury classification, neurologic prognostication, and bowel and bladder management.

Key Principles

- The anorectal exam reflects neurologic function of the S4–S5 spinal segments.
- The sensory exam includes assessment of light touch, and sharp/dull discrimination of the skin just lateral to the anal mucocutaneous junction. This point is the key sensory point for the S4 and S5 dermatomes.
- Deep pressure sensation is tested by digital rectal exam.
- The motor rectal exam identifies the presence or absence of voluntary external anal sphincter contraction; there is no quantitative evaluation as with other muscles.
- Reflex examination includes the bulbocavernosus and anocutaneous reflexes.

Indications

- The rectal exam should be performed on all spinal injured individuals as part of their comprehensive assessment.

Contraindications

- Perineal trauma
- Pre-existing anorectal pathology

Special Considerations

- The individual should be alert and able to understand and respond to the examiner's directions to fully assess neurologic function, though reflex function can be assessed in an individual with disorders of consciousness.

Key Procedural Steps

- The anorectal examination after new SCI is performed as the final part of the neurologic assessment to minimize spine movement.
- The individual should be log-rolled into a side-lying position.
- The sensory exam of the S3 key point, located over the ischial tuberosities, is conveniently performed in this position.
- Perform the light touch examination of the S4–S5 dermatome as with all other dermatomes of the body. Record the result.
- Perform the sharp/dull assessment of the S4–S5 dermatome as with all other dermatomes. Record the result.
- Perform an internal rectal examination.
- If the light touch and pinprick exams of S4–S5 revealed no preserved sensation, assess the individual for deep pressure sensation during the internal exam.
- Perform the motor exam by asking the individual to squeeze the sphincter muscle around the examiner's finger. Record the presence or absence of voluntary muscle contraction.
- Assess for the bulbocavernosus reflex by gently pulling on the indwelling catheter, while the finger is still inserted in the rectum. The reflex is present when the anal sphincter contracts in response to this stimulus.

Anticipated Problems

- Pressure sensation is only indicative of preserved sensation when it occurs in the S4–S5 dermatome. It is not assessed for any other dermatome.
- If it is unsafe to place the individual in side-lying, an abbreviated anorectal exam can be performed in supine.
- Do not ask the individual to bear down as part of the motor exam. Performing a Valsalva maneuver may yield a false positive result.
- If there is no indwelling catheter, the bulbocavernosus reflex may be elicited by gently squeezing the glans penis of a man or stimulating the clitoris of a woman.
- Voluntary contraction of the sphincter may be confused with a reflex response. Examiner experience is helpful in differentiating the two.

Helpful Hints

- Verbal preparation for the anorectal exam is critical to maximize an individual's comfort. Anxiety about this exam may yield inaccurate results if the individual contracts the sphincter muscle because of anxiety.

■ The results of the sensorimotor and sacral reflex exams are an excellent indicator and predictor of future bowel, bladder, and sexual function and can be very helpful in planning optimal bowel and bladder management.

Suggested Readings

Instep International Standards Training E Program. American Spinal Injury Association. http://www.torranceinc.com/clients/asia/

Marino RJ, Barros T, Biering-Sorensen, et al. International standards for neurological classification of spinal cord injury. *J Spinal Cord Med.* 2003; 26(Suppl 1):S50–S56.

Neurologic Examination: Sensory Testing

Adam B. Stein MD

Description

An examination to determine the most caudal level of preserved sensation as well as the presence and location of any other pinprick (PP) or light touch (LT) sensation below the level of SCI.

Key Principles

- Examine 28 dermatomes on each side of the body from C2 to S4/S5.
- One key sensory point represents each dermatome.
- LT and PP are the two modalities that are required for testing.
- LT reflects afferent transmission in the dorsal columns.
- PP reflects afferent transmission in spinothalamic tracts.
- Each dermatome is scored either 0, 1, or 2 for absent, impaired, or normal sensation, respectively.
- The maximum sensory score is 56 for each side of the body or 112 total.
- The sensory level is defined as the most caudal level that tests normally for both LT and PP.
- Testing of other sensory modalities does not affect determination of the sensory level.

Indications/Contraindications

- Examinee must awake and be able to understand instructions and respond to examiners questions.

Special Considerations

- Performing the sensory examination 72 hours after injury allows the examiner to perform an accurate exam in the vast majority of cases.

Key Procedural Steps

- The examination is performed with the individual supine.
- Perform the light touch examination using a wisp of cotton.
- Demonstrate normal sensation by lightly stroking an unaffected part of the body such as the cheek.
- Begin at the C2 sensory point and progress caudally through the S4/S5 key point.

- For each point, ask the individual to indicate when they feel a touch sensation.
- Score the dermatome 0 if the stimulus is not felt at least 80% of the time.
- If the stimulus is felt at least 80% of the time, score the dermatome a 2 if it feels the same as on the cheek and a 1 if it feels different.
- Perform the PP examination with a safety pin.
- Demonstrate sharp sensation by pricking the cheek with the sharp end.
- Demonstrate dull sensation by touching the cheek with the rounded end.
- Begin at the C2 sensory point and progress caudally to S4/S5.
- At least 80% correct responses indicate that sharp/dull discrimination is present.
- Score the dermatome a 2 if the sharp sensation feels the same as on the face and 1 if it feels different.

Anticipated Problems

- When there appears to be sensation present at T3, when there is no sensation at T1, T2, or T4, the sensation is likely attributable to the C4 dermatome, which descends onto the upper chest, and the T3 dermatome should be scored zero.
- Do not confuse the ability to feel pressure with the patient's ability to discriminate sharp from dull.
- The individual only is credited with pin sensation if they can discriminate sharp from dull.
- Hyperesthesia is not normal; if the individual reports that the sharp side of the pin gives an abnormally noxious sensation, the sensation is impaired and scored as 1.
- If the individual reports that both sharp and dull end of the pin cause a sharp sensation, the score is zero for that dermatome as the patient cannot tell the two apart.

Helpful Hints

- When a key sensory point is unavailable for testing, use another area within that dermatome if available. If no such area available, score the dermatome "NT" for not testable.
- Ensure that the individual's vision is blocked during testing.

- Utilize only one stimulation to elicit a response from a patient. Utilizing multiple, consecutive sensory stimuli may produce a false positive response.
- Discourage guessing.
- Alter the order and cadence of stimuli.
- Beware of mitigating circumstances, which may result in inaccurate testing, such as severe pain or cognitive deficit.

Suggested Readings

Marino RJ, Barros T, Biering-Sorensen, et al. International standards for neurological classification of spinal cord injury. *J Spinal Cord Med.* 2003; 26(Suppl 1):S50–S6.

American Spinal Injury Association. *Reference Manual for the International Standards for Neurological Classification of Spinal Cord Injury.* Chicago: American Spinal Injury Association; 2003:7–20.

Section II: Interventions

Neurologic Examination: Sensory Testing, Dermatomes

Thomas N. Bryce MD

Description
Assess for pinprick (PP) and light touch (LT) sensory abnormalities in all dermatomes.

Key Principles
- Sensation for LT and PP is graded: 0, 1, 2, and not testable (NT).
- NT is used when the key points are unavailable for testing or sensation over the face is abnormal.

Light touch
- Grade 0 (absent): Individual does not reliably report being touched.
- Grade 1 (impaired): Individual correctly reports being touched but the touch is different than that where sensation is normal, ie, the face.
- Grade 2 (normal): The sensation is exactly the same as the face.

Pinprick
- Grade 0 (absent): Individual does not reliably distinguish between the sharp and dull ends of a safety pin.
- Grade 1 (impaired): Individual reliably distinguishes between the sharp and dull ends of a safety pin but the intensity of the sharpness is different than on the face.
- Grade 2 (normal): The individual reliably distinguishes between sharp and dull and the intensity of PP is exactly the same as the face.

Indications
- Perform on all individuals with SCI.

Special Considerations
- Perform with the individual supine.

Key Procedural Steps

Key sensory points
- C2: One centimeter lateral to the occipital protuberance at the base of the skull.
- An alternate key point for C2 is at least 3 cm behind the ear.
- C3: At the apex of the supraclavicular fossa
- C4: Over the acromioclavicular joint
- C5: On the lateral (radial) side of the antecubital fossa just proximal to the elbow
- C6: On the dorsal surface of the proximal phalanx of the thumb
- C7: On the dorsal surface of the proximal phalanx of the middle finger
- C8: On the dorsal surface of the proximal phalanx of the little finger
- T1: On the medial (ulnar) side of the antecubital fossa, just proximal to the medial epicondyle of the humerus
- T2: At the apex of the axilla
- T3: At the midclavicular line and the third intercostal space, found by palpating the anterior chest to locate the third rib and the corresponding third intercostal space below it
- T4: At the midclavicular line and the fourth intercostal space, located at the level of the nipples
- T5: At the midclavicular line and the fifth intercostal space, located midway between the level of the nipples and the level of the xiphisternum
- T6: At the midclavicular line, located at the level of the xiphisternum
- T7: At the midclavicular line, located at one quarter the distance between the level of the xiphisternum and the level of the umbilicus
- T8: At the midclavicular line, located at one half the distance between the level of the xiphisternum and the level of the umbilicus
- T9: At the midclavicular line, located at three quarters of the distance between the level of the xiphisternum and the level of the umbilicus
- T10: At the midclavicular line, located at the level of the umbilicus
- T11: At the midclavicular line, midway between the level of the umbilicus and the inguinal ligament
- T12: At the midclavicular line, over the midpoint of the inguinal ligament
- L1: Midway between the key sensory points for T12 and L2
- L2: On the anterior medial thigh, midway on a line between the midpoint of the inguinal ligament and the medial femoral condyle above the knee
- L3: At the medial femoral condyle above the knee

- L4: Over the medial malleolus
- L5: On the dorsum of the foot at the third metatarsal phalangeal joint
- S1: On the lateral side of the heel
- S2: In the popliteal fossa of the knee at the midpoint
- S3: Over the ischial tuberosity
- S4/S5: In the perianal area, less than 1 cm lateral to the mucocutaneous junction

Anticipated Problems

- Testing for T3 too rostrally may actually be testing the C4 dermatome.

Helpful Hints

- Frequently retest the face to allow the individual to maintain a frame of reference for normal.
- Try and trick the individual by moving the stimulus next to the skin without actually touching it to see if the individual is guessing.

Suggested Reading

American Spinal Injury Association. *Reference Manual for the International Standards for Neurological Classification of Spinal Cord Injury.* Chicago: American Spinal Injury Association; 2003:7–20.

Pharmacologic and Thermal Treatment of Acute Spinal Cord Injury

Igor Rakovchik DO

Description

Various pharmacologic agents and thermal techniques have been administered after acute SCI with the intent of improving neurologic outcomes with limited success.

Key Principles

- The primary mechanism for traumatic SCI is typically mechanical, with shearing and/or compression of neural tissue.
- Secondary mechanisms of SCI involve inflammation, ischemia, and axonal degeneration.
- Pharmacologic treatments have focused primarily on limiting the impact of the secondary mechanisms of SCI.
- Hypothermia is thought to have several neuroprotective effects such as enzymatic slowing and decreasing cellular energy expenditure.
- Systemic or local hypothermia has not been shown to have a consistent neuroprotective benefit in animal studies in acute SCI.
- There is currently insufficient evidence to advocate the use of local or systemic hypothermia in human subjects.

Pharmacologic treatments

Pharmacologic treatments or neuroprotectants that have been studied in large randomized placebo-controlled trials include methylprednisolone (MP), ganglioside (GM-1), tirilazad, and naloxone.

- Methylprednisolone
  - MP is a synthetic glucocorticoid, the primary action of which is believed to be lipid peroxidation.
  - MP was studied in three large randomized clinical trials, the National Acute Spinal Cord Injury Studies (NASCIS)
  - The functional significance of the outcomes and the methodology and data analysis of the NASCIS studies have generated controversy.
  - In NASCIS II, neurologic improvements were reported to occur when MP was administered within 8 hours of injury.
  - In NASCIS III, the best outcomes were reported to occur if MP was given within 3 hours of injury for

24 hours or within 3 to 8 hours after injury for 48 hours.

- Ganglioside
  - GM-1 is thought to impact neuronal plasticity and repair mechanisms, particularly in preventing apoptosis and promoting neuronal sprouting.
  - GM-1 has been studied as an adjunct treatment after administration of MP, but has not been shown to have a significant clinical benefit.
- Tirilazad is an inhibitor of lipid peroxidation and has been shown to have neuroprotective effects in animal SCI models.
- Naloxone is an opioid receptor antagonist is thought to reduce tissue infarction, neutrophil accumulation, and chemokine expression in rat studies.
- Gacyclidine is a noncompetitive NMDA antagonist that has been studied experimentally in rats.

Indications

- No clinical evidence exists to definitely recommend the use of any neuroprotective pharmacologic agent in the treatment of acute SCI to improve functional recovery at this time.
- Historically, high-dose MP administration has been thought to be the standard of care for the pharmacological treatment of acute SCI if given within 8 hours of traumatic SCI.
- No clinical evidence exists to recommend cooling.

Contraindications

Methylprednisolone

- Penetrating trauma such as gunshot or stab wounds due to the theoretical risk of infection
- Isolated cauda equina or nerve root injury
- Pregnancy

Special Considerations

- Discontinue the administration of MP as soon as possible in neurologically intact patients or in those in whom prior neurologic symptoms have resolved.

Key Procedural Steps

Methylprednisolone

- Confirm time since injury is <8 hours.
- Administer a bolus dose 30 mg/kg body weight over 1 hour.
- Administer a 5.4 mg/kg/h maintenance dose for 23 hours if the injury occurred within 3 hours prior to initial dose.
- Administer a 5.4 mg/kg/h maintenance dose for 48 hours if the injury occurred 3 to 8 hours prior to initial dose.
- Note: Begin intravenous maintenance dose 45 minutes after conclusion of initial bolus.

Anticipated Problems

- Increased incidence of wound infection and sepsis
- Increased incidence and severity of respiratory complications
- Increased incidence of pulmonary embolism
- Increased incidence of GI bleeding and pancreatitis
- Steroids may mask abdominal signs of hollow viscous injury.

Helpful Hints

- The use of steroids remains a recommendation and not a universal standard of care.
- The use of steroids in patients with penetrating wounds may have adverse complications and worsen outcome.

Suggested Readings

Bracken MB. Steroids for acute spinal cord injury (update). *Cochrane Database Syst Rev.* 2007; (2):CD001046.

Consortium for spinal cord medicine et al. Early acute management in adults with spinal cord injury: a clinical practice guideline for heath-care professionals. *J Spinal Cord Med.* 2008;31(4):403–479.

Kwon BK, Mann C, Sohn HM, et al. Hypothermia for spinal cord injury. *Spine J.* 2008;8(6):859–874.

Pulmonary Management: Glossopharyngeal Breathing

Thomas N. Bryce MD

Description
Gulps of air propelled with the glossopharyngeal muscles past the glottis into the lungs can increase the amount of air in the lungs. This is called glossopharyngeal breathing (GPB), air stacking, or frog breathing.

Key Principles
- As first described by Dail for persons affected by poliomyelitis, gulping air into the lungs can increase lung volumes.
- The glottis closes with each gulp.
- One breath usually consists of six to nine gulps of 40 to 200 mL each.
- A proficient glossopharyngeal breather will average approximately eight or nine breaths per minute, with each breath requiring 12 to 15 gulps.
- An increased amount of air in the lungs can improve oxygen delivery.
- When this increased amount of air is expelled with a cough, cough flow is increased, increasing the ability to clear secretions.
- When this increased amount of air is expelled in a controlled fashion during speech, the volume of the speech can be increased.
- Use of assisted cough in conjunction with GPB can increase the cough flows to an extent much greater than when either technique is used alone.

Indications
- Persons with little or no diaphragm strength who wish to breathe free of electrical stimulation or mechanical ventilation for limited periods
- Persons who need help eliminating secretions due to a weak cough
- Persons at risk for atelectasis and pneumonia due to a low vital capacity

Contraindications
- Inability to tolerate a partially or fully deflated tracheostomy tube cuff
- Inability to tolerate either plugging of or placement of a one-way valve on a tracheostomy tube

Special Considerations
- The presence of midbrain damage can impair the ability to perform the technique as glottic closure and opening required for gulping air and coughing depends on contraction of laryngeal muscles.

Key Procedural Steps
- Instruct individual to take in a deep breath.
- Without individual exhaling, have the individual take in as many large gulps as they can, propelling air using the muscles of the tongue, soft palate, pharynx, and larynx.
- The glottis should audibly close with each gulp.
- In order to cough when no more air can be accommodated, individual should be instructed to cough.
- Alternatively, in order to expire normally when no more air can be accommodated, individual should be instructed to allow passive exhalation.

Anticipated Problems
- GPB is less often successful in those with a tracheostomy tube.
- It will not work if there is a significant air leak below the glottis such as is the case with an uncapped tracheostomy or even a capped one if gulped air can escape around the outer walls of the tube and out the stoma.

Helpful Hints
- Remind individual not to swallow air.
- Monitor the efficiency of GPB by spirometrically measuring the milliliters of air per gulp, gulps per breath, and breaths per minute.
- Gulp efficiency can be defined as: (MVGPB – VC)/NGMI, where MVGPB is the maximum volume that could be gulped in, VC is the vital capacity, and NGMI is the number of gulps to a maximum insufflation.
- During training, the nostrils can be sealed to demonstrate the need for the soft palate to seal off the nasopharynx.

Suggested Readings

Bach JR. New approaches in the rehabilitation of the traumatic high level quadriplegic. *Am J Phys Med Rehabil.* 1991;70:13–20.

Bach JR, Alba AS. Noninvasive options for ventilatory support of the traumatic high level quadriplegic. *Chest.* 1990;98:613–619.

Dail CW. Glossopharyngeal breathing by paralyzed patients. *Calif Med.* 1951;75:15–25.

Kirby NA, Barnerias MJ, Siebens AA. An evaluation of assisted cough in quadriparetic patients. *Arch Phys Med Rehabil.* 1966;47:705–710.

Webber B, Higgens J. *Glossopharyngeal Breathing: What, When and How?* (video). Holbrook, England: Aslan Studios; 1999.

Section II: Interventions

Pulmonary Management: Phrenic Nerve and Diaphragm Pacing

Thomas N. Bryce MD ■ Kristjan T. Ragnarsson MD

Description

Phrenic nerve and diaphragm pacing are techniques whereupon the diaphragm can be stimulated allowing nonmechanical ventilation in a person without spontaneous diaphragm motor function. Phrenic nerve and diaphragm pacing both allow better speech, mobility, and cosmesis than mechanical ventilation.

Key Principles

Phrenic nerve pacing

- Stimulating cuffs are placed around both phrenic nerves in the chest or neck.
- Phrenic nerve pacing requires thoracotomy.
- Fully implantable system in that there are no wires protruding through the skin.
- Stimulator is implanted under skin on anterior chest wall.
- Implanted wires connect electrodes to stimulator.
- Control unit and batteries are external.
- Radiofrequency control signals are transmitted via antenna.
- Stimulation is started 2 weeks postoperatively.
- Reconditioning of diaphragm may take 2 to 3 months.

Diaphragm pacing

- Electrodes are placed directly into diaphragm through a laparoscopic approach.
- Diaphragm pacing does not require thoracotomy.
- Stimulating leads extend outside abdomen and attach to stimulator unit, control unit, and batteries, which are external.
- Stimulation can be begun immediately after implantation.
- Reconditioning of diaphragm to a degree that a ventilator is no longer needed can take several months although it has been accomplished in as early as 1 week.

Indications

- High-level SCI with ventilator dependence

Contraindications

- Nonintact phrenic nerves

- Diseased lungs that would not be able to sustain adequate respiration if neuromuscular control was regained through placement of a pacing system

Special Considerations

- Performed in specialized centers.
- Strong motivation and support is needed for conditioning.
- Available professional technical knowledge is essential.
- Current technology is unable to provide co-ordination of respiratory drive and pacing.
- Current technology is unable to match ventilation and metabolic demand.
- Current technology is unable to provide effective cough.

Key Procedural Steps

Implantation

- Consider indications and contraindications.
- Verify viability of phrenic nerves by surface electrical stimulation and fluoroscopy.
- Ensure healthy lungs and airways.
- Identify specialized center with capability to implant system.

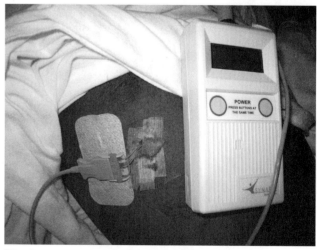

Diaphragm pacer wires attached to pacer.

- Diaphragm pacer wires are typically implanted using an abdominal laparoscopic approach and may be performed as same day surgery.

Weaning use of diaphragm pacer
- Perform pulmonary hygiene.
- Program the respiratory rate, stimulus amplitude, pulse width, inspiration interval, pulse frequency, and pulse ramp modulation on pacer for all the electrode leads using a programming device.
- Programming typically needs to be done only once.
- Attach external pacer to the wire connector exiting from the chest wall.
- Activate pacer.
- Remove patient from ventilator and place on trach collar or T-piece.
- Obtain vital capacity while being paced.
- Monitor for clinical signs of respiratory muscle fatigue, for example, elevated heart rate, elevated rating of perceived exertion.
- Monitor the end tidal CO_2 to provide objective evidence of respiratory muscle fatigue.
- Replace on ventilator support and turn off pacer if there are signs of fatigue.
- Rest at least 1 hour.

- Repeat process, simultaneously increasing the duration of pacing as tolerated.

Anticipated Problems
- Mechanical system may fail so a backup ventilator is needed.
- There is a risk of phrenic nerve injury with placement of phrenic electrodes.

Helpful Hints
- Consider implantation of diaphragm pacing system in the early phase of SCI to help shorten the time on a ventilator in those who are expected to have difficulty weaning from the ventilator.
- Diaphragm pacing can be performed on the ventilator to provide conditioning if anxiety limits use of a trach collar or T-piece.
- Treatment of anxiety is essential to successful weaning.

Suggested Readings
Glenn WWL, Hogan JF, Loke JSO, et al. Ventilatory support by pacing of the conditioned diaphragm in quadriplegia. *N Engl J Med.* 1984;310:1150–1155.

Onders RP, Elmo MJ, Ignagni AR. Diaphragm pacing stimulation system for tetraplegia in individuals injured during childhood or adolescence. *J Spinal Cord Med.* 2007; 30(Suppl 1):S25–S29.

Section II: Interventions

Pulmonary Management: Secretion Removal

Thomas N. Bryce MD

Description

Techniques that can be used to facilitate clearing the airway of excess secretions include assisted coughing, suctioning, use of an insufflator-exsufflator, therapeutic chest percussion, postural drainage, and bronchoscopy. Medications can also be used to alter the consistency of the secretions, facilitating their removal.

Key Principles

Assisted cough

- A cough performed in conjunction with a rostrally directed abdominal thrust (usually performed by another person).

Suctioning

- Generally performed through tracheostomy tube or endotracheal tube.
- Superficially performed for secretions in proximal airway distal to and within tracheal tube.
- Deeply performed for secretions in main stem bronchus near carina.
- Directional catheters available to reach problematic side

Insufflator-exsufflator

- An electrically powered external mechanical device, which can provide positive pressure and negative pressure to the airway in succession
- Rate of flow, duration of flow, and applied pressures can be adjusted.
- Simulates a cough

Postural drainage

- Facilitates drainage from individual lobes
- Combinations of prone, supine, head elevated, head lowered (Trandelenberg), right side up, and left side up positions allow all lobes to be drained.

Chest percussion

- Perform in conjunction with postural drainage.
- Use cupped hand or mechanical device.

Bronchoscopy

- Perform on or off ventilator.
- Allows visualization and directed removal of excess secretions.

Medications

- Nebulized acetylcysteine or sodium bicarbonate can loosen or solubilize thick mucus.
- Hydration can loosen secretions thickened by dehydration.
- Guaifenesin taken orally can also loosen secretions.

Indications

- Perform when secretion clearance is not adequate for amount of secretions that are present.
- Facilitate weaning off a ventilator.
- Prevent mucus plugging, atelectasis, and pneumonia.

Contraindications

- Avoid head-down postural drainage if there is high risk for reflux or emesis, such as during tube feed administration.
- Avoid insufflation-exsufflation in presence of pneumothorax.

Special Considerations

- Perform techniques and administer medication around the clock, as needed.
- Typically begin at 4-hour intervals for chest percussion, postural drainage, and nebulizer administration.
- Rotating beds that allow positioning for postural drainage with rotation can decrease the staff burden.

Key Procedural Steps

Assisted cough

- Place the base of the assistant's hand over the upper abdomen just below the ribcage (two hands may be needed for smaller assistants).
- On a prearranged count coordinate a cough by the individual needing one with an upwardly directed abdominal force by the assistant.
- Repeat as necessary.

160

Suctioning

- Insert suction catheter gently down trachea until resistance is felt (deep suction).
- While steadily pulling out catheter, simultaneously twist catheter and intermittently place finger over air vent to provide intermittent suction.
- Repeat as necessary.

Insufflator-exsufflator

- Attach insufflator-exsufflator tubing to tracheostomy tube.
- Perform exsufflation (apply negative pressure) with pressure between −40 and −70 cm H_2O for 2 to 3 seconds.
- Perform insufflation (apply positive pressure) with pressure of 40 cm H_2O for 1 to 2 seconds.
- Follow insufflation by exsufflation.
- Repeat as necessary.

Postural drainage

- Sequentially position head elevated, head lowered (Trandelenberg), right side up, and left side up, both prone and supine.

Chest percussion

- Perform in conjunction with postural drainage.

- Using a cupped hand vigorously strike the individual over the draining lobes.

Anticipated Problems

- Chest percussion is ineffective if not performed vigorously.
- Failure to perform techniques in a person with ineffective cough usually leads to plugging of airways by mucus and secondary atelectasis, pneumonia, and pleural effusions.

Helpful Hints

- Adding on an inline suction attachment to insuffator-exsuffator tracheostomy tube attachment can allow for removal of exsufflated secretions from tubing or tracheostomy tube before they are insufflated back down the bronchial tree into the lungs.

Suggested Readings

Bryce TN, Ragnarsson KT, Stein AS. Spinal cord injury. In: Braddom RL, ed. *Physical Medicine and Rehabilitation*. 3rd ed. Philadelphia: Saunders Elsevier; 2007:1285–1389.

Consortium for Spinal Cord Medicine. Respiratory management following spinal cord injury: a clinical practice guideline for health-care professionals. *J Spinal Cord Med.* 2005;28(3):259–293.

Section II: Interventions

Pulmonary Management: Ventilator Management

Melvin S. Mejia MD

Description

Mechanical ventilatory support is initiated whenever a person is unable to maintain effective gas exchange, compromising survival.

Key Principles

- Early tracheostomy and ventilatory support is suggested for those with complete injuries above C5.
- Measurements of the vital capacity (VC) and the negative inspiratory force (NIF) provide an assessment of inspiratory muscle strength and ability to clear secretions.
- Deterioration of VC (normal 65 to 75 mL/kg) can result from atelectasis and mucus plugging.
- Individuals with a NIF value more negative than -30 cm H_2O are more likely to be successfully weaned than those with values less negative than -20 cm H_2O.
- Using tidal volumes (TV) of >12 to 15 mL/kg IBW can facilitate resolution of atelectasis and shorten time on the ventilator.
- The risk for barotrauma is increased if peak airway pressure (pressure required to deliver the TV) is persistently above 40 cm H_2O.
- Assist control ventilation (ACV) is the mode most commonly recommended.
- The ACV mode minimizes an individual's effort by providing full mechanical support with every breath, and is often the mode chosen because it provides the greatest degree of support.
- Progressive ventilator-free breathing (PVFB) (using the T-piece or trach collar) is the preferred ventilator weaning method for persons with respiratory failure due to SCI-related bellows weakness.
- PVFB allows a deconditioned diaphragm full interval rests between weaning trials, enhancing verbal communication during the rests, and providing a safety interval for ventilator disconnection in those who may not be ultimately fully weanable.

Indications

Indications for mechanical ventilation

- Apnea and physical signs of respiratory distress (cyanosis, accessory muscle use, tachypnea, tachycardia, diaphoresis, altered mental status, hypotension, hypertension)
- Impending respiratory failure: $PaCO_2$ >50 mm Hg, PaO_2 <50 mm Hg, pH <7.30
- Severe hypoxemia unresponsive to high oxygen delivery (PaO_2 <50 mm Hg, FiO_2 >0.6)
- Downward trend of the VC (<15 mL/kg IBW)
- Inability to handle secretions

Special Considerations

Essential respiratory care

- Positioning
- Percussion
- Aggressive secretion removal
- Respiratory exercises
- Bronchodilators, mucolytics

Key Procedural Steps

Ventilator setup

- Calculate ideal body weight (IBW)
- Mode: ACV; TV: 12 to 15 mL/kg; rate: 12/min; sigh 300 to 500 mL >TV; flow rate 70 L/min; titrate O_2 to sat >92%.
- Increase TV by 50 to 100 mL/day (max 25 mL/kg IBW) and peak flow by 10 L/min daily (max 120 L/min) as long as peak airway pressure is <40 cm H_2O.
- Taper positive end-expiratory pressure (PEEP) to zero.
- Check VC, NIF, arterial blood gas, chest X-ray to monitor for adequacy of ventilation and management of atelectasis.

Conditions for initiation of weaning

- Afebrile with stable vital signs >24 hours
- VC preferably at least 15 mL/kg of IBW (1.0 to 1.2 L)
- NIF preferably more than -24 cm H_2O
- FiO2 preferably 0.21
- pH 7.35 to 7.45, PCO_2 >35 to 45 mm Hg, PaO_2 >75 mm Hg
- Respiratory rate <25/min
- Manageable secretions, CXR clear
- Hemodynamically stable, cooperative individual

Weaning

- Initiate PVFB with the initial trial at 15 to 30 minutes twice a day.
- Measure pre- and post-trial VC, which helps identify presence of muscle fatigue (>20% drop).
- Increase trials by 1 hour increments twice a day as individual tolerates until completely off the ventilator.
- Passy-Muir valve used during the trial to allow for vocalization
- Once off the ventilator for 24 to 48 hours using the Passy-Muir valve, start tracheostomy plugging and increase duration as tolerated.

Conditions for discontinuation of weaning

- Drop in VC >20%
- Heart rate >20 beats from baseline
- Respirations >10 breaths from baseline
- Blood pressure ±30 mm Hg from baseline
- Oxygen saturation <92% with FiO_2 >20% higher than ordered
- Evidence of infection, temperature >101, fatigue

Anticipated Problems

- Ventilator-associated pneumonia
- Ventilator-induced diaphragmatic dysfunction
- Barotrauma and bronchopleural fistula
- Oxygen toxicity

Helpful Hints

- Tailor the weaning process to the individual, keeping in mind that the end result is more important than the speed in which the methods are done.
- The importance of vaccinations and remaining a non-smoker cannot be overemphasized.

Suggested Readings

Berly M. Respiratory management during the first five days after spinal cord injury. *J Spinal Cord Med.* 2007;30:309–318.

Brown R, DiMarco A. Respiratory dysfunction and management in spinal cord injury. *Resp Care.* 2006;51(8):853–870.

Epstein S. Complications associated with mechanical ventilation. In: Tobin M, ed. *Principles and Practice of Mechanical Ventilation*, 2nd ed. McGraw Hill, Inc. 2006;877–1032.

Marino P. Discontinuing mechanical ventilation. In: Marino P, (ed). *The ICU Book*. 3rd ed. Lippincott Williams and Wilkins. 2006;511–527.

Restorative Therapies: Body Weight Supported Ambulation

Kristjan T. Ragnarsson MD

Description

A person with SCI is placed in a harness, which permits lower limb movements, and is suspended from an overhead beam over a treadmill. Ambulation training is performed by varying the amount of body weight support (BWS) and the speed of the treadmill with a therapist guiding and setting the lower limbs properly.

Key Principles

- Builds on reflex or voluntary activation of lower limb muscles
- Improves ambulation skills in persons with incomplete SCI, similar to other methods of ambulation training
- May have therapeutic benefits similar to functional electrical stimulation (FES) ergometry
- May be combined with other forms of therapeutic technology, for example, FES and robotics
- The amount of BWS is dependent on the co-ordination, balance, strength, and function of the individual.
- Activities other than walking can be facilitated with BWS, for example, crawling training for pediatric patients and balance training in sitting or standing.

Indications

- To improve ambulation skills of nonambulatory persons with neurologically incomplete SCI
- To obtain the therapeutic benefits of actively exercising paralyzed lower limbs
- To facilitate axonal regeneration and circuitry in combination with experimental treatments

Contraindications

- Unstable cardiovascular conditions
- Severe osteoporosis with pathological fractures
- Significant pathology of lower limb joints
- Extensive lumbosacral LMN damage
- Excessive lower limb spasticity
- Severe lower limb joint contractures

Special Considerations

- Functional benefits (ambulation) achieved only in patients with incomplete SCI or some lower extremity motor function
- Therapeutic benefits obtained with regular and continuous application
- Expensive equipment
- Manpower demanding therapy

Key Procedural Steps

- Perform detailed neurologic examination.
- Set specific and realistic goals.
- Select motivated and compliant participants.
- Place individual in harness within suspending apparatus over treadmill or the ground with the chest and shoulders centered over the hips.
- Adjust the four overhead straps on the harness so that the individual is standing upright with the knees slightly flexed and the ankles in neutral position on the ground or treadmill.
- If the torso is leaning forward, tighten the front straps to realign.
- If the torso is leaning backward, tighten the back straps to realign.
- If the trunk is leaning to one side, tighten the front and back straps on that side to realign.
- Once the treadmill is moving, if the heel is not contacting the treadmill during heel strike, loosen all four straps a little at a time until this occurs.
- Initially provide BWS to the point where gait is as normal as possible.
- Initially set the treadmill speed at <0.5 mph to facilitate a proper gait pattern.
- For severely impaired persons, the legs should be moved manually by the therapist to establish a proper gait pattern.
- Ensure there is adequate hip extension during terminal stance in order to stretch the hip flexors to trigger the spinal cord central pattern generator.
- Manually control the trunk or use a pelvic harness that constrains the pelvis in order to eliminate backward pelvic rotation or forward trunk lean, which can inhibit hip extension.

- Initially limit sessions to three repetitions of 3 minutes of walking followed by a 5-minute rest or until the gait appears to deteriorate.
- Gradually increase walking duration by 30 to 60 seconds per trial.
- Perform one half to one hour sessions 2 to 4 times per week.
- If no improvement is made over a 2- to 3-week period, the therapy time may be better spent on other activities.
- Progress patient by either reducing the amount of BWS or increasing the treadmill speed.

Anticipated Problems
- Insufficient insurance benefits
- Mild knee injuries

Helpful Hints
- Has not been shown to benefit persons with neurologically complete and flaccid paralysis of lower limbs
- To facilitate hip extension one may place a ball between the patient's pelvis and a restraining barrier in front of the patient forcing the patient to maintain his or her pelvis in an anterior position.

Suggested Readings
Dobkin BH, Apple D, Barbeau H, et al. Methods for a randomized trial of weight-supported treadmill training versus conventional training for walking during inpatient rehabilitation after incomplete traumatic spinal cord injury. *Neurorehabil Neural Repair.* 2003;17(3):153–167.

Protocols for Partial Weight Bearing, Gait and Balance Therapy. Tempe: Mobility Research Education Department.

Restorative Therapies: Functional Electrical Stimulation

Kristjan T. Ragnarsson MD

Description

The application of electrical currents to neural tissue in order to restore a degree of control to abnormal or absent body functions

Key Principles

- The LMN must be intact.
- The strength of the functional electrical stimulation (FES) induced muscle contraction must be forceful, controllable, and repeatable.
- The electrical stimulus must not be painful.
- The neural structures must not be damaged by the FES.
- The method of FES delivery must be acceptable to the user.
- The FES may use either surface or implanted electrodes.

Indications

Upper limb FES for function

- Allow palmar and lateral prehension and perhaps arm reach for persons with C5–C6 tetraplegia with intact C7 and C8 LMN.

Lower limb FES for function (when available)

- Allow standing with a walker and bilateral ankle-foot orthoses (AFO)
- Allow reaching above shoulder with one hand
- Allow swing-to or swing-through gait
- Allow better trunk control and sitting position

Bladder, bowel, and sexual function FES

- Allow control of the bladder and bowel, erections, and ejaculation for persons with neurologically complete suprasacral SCI with intact sacral LMN and documented problems with other forms of bladder management.

Phrenic and diaphragmic pacing

- Allow independence in breathing for those who are ventilator-dependent.

FES ergometry

- Cardiovascular conditioning
- Improve serum lipid profile

- Decrease fat infiltration between muscle fibers
- Decrease serum glucose
- Improve glucose utilization
- Decrease leg edema and acrocyanosis
- Potentially reduce deep vein thrombosis incidence
- Increase bulk, strength, and endurance of paralyzed muscles.
- Potentially prevent and facilitate healing of pressure ulcers.
- Potentially reverse osteoporosis (10% to 30%).
- Improve depression scores, self-image, and perceived appearance.
- Facilitate neuroplasticity by increasing secretion of nerve growth factors, brain-derived neurotrophic factor (BDNF), and endorphins.

Contraindications

- Muscles paralyzed by LMN damage
- Cardiac pacemaker/defibrillator (implanted)
- Heart disease (dysrhythmia, congestive heart failure)
- Pregnancy
- Severe spasticity
- Severe joint contractures
- Severe osteoporosis with pathological fractures

Special Considerations

FES for upper limbs

- Deliver current via surface electrodes combined with wrist-hand orthosis; percutaneous electrodes and wires; or implanted electrodes, wires, and stimulator (Freehand).
- Availability of implanted systems has historically been very limited due to limited commercial demand.

FES for lower limbs

- Success toward effective ambulation has been limited due to high-energy expenditure, slow speed of gait, poor balance, insufficient exercise response in high SCI, and inadequate system designs.
- A system with surface electrodes for bilateral quadriceps and gluteus muscles and the peroneal nerves with an external control unit and batteries (Parastep) is available but rarely used.

- Under development is a system with implanted intramuscular electrodes with an eight-channel stimulator and connecting wires, but with an external control unit, batteries, and programming station (VA/CWRU Standing System).

FES for bladder, bowel, and sexual function

- Stimulation of anterior sacral nerve roots causes bladder contraction and urination.
- For the Finetech-Brindley system described below, reports indicate successful urination on demand and continence between stimulations in 80% to 90%, increased bladder capacity, fewer episodes of infections, and successful defecation achieved by adjusting stimulus parameters.
- Electrical stimulation may generate erection and ejaculation, but is considered inferior to use of medications and vibrations, respectively.
- Availability is limited.

Key Procedural Steps

FES for bladder, bowel, and sexual function

- Implant electrodes bilaterally on the S2–S4 anterior nerve roots extradurally by sacral laminectomy (Finetech-Brindley system).
- Perform posterior sacral rhizotomy through a T11–L2 laminectomy to secure continence.

- Implant a receiver-stimulator on the anterior abdominal wall.
- Program the external control unit

FES ergometry

- Image lower extremity joints and long bones to assess for fracture, dislocation, osteopenia, and heterotopic ossification
- Check to see that there is adequate ROM in the affected joints of the extremity to be exercised in the ergometer
- Place on ergometer, apply electrodes, and begin session
- Continue therapy sessions 2 to 3 times per week

Anticipated Problems

- Mechanical failures
- Infected implanted devices (rare)
- Pathologic limb fracture from ergometry is rare

Helpful Hints

- Clinical usefulness may increase with development of miniature modular FES systems, which are totally implantable by endoscopic procedures.

Suggested Reading

Ragnarsson KT. Functional electrical stimulation after spinal cord injury: current use, therapeutic effects and future directions. *Spinal Cord.* 2008;46:255–274.

Sexuality and Reproduction: Electroejaculation and Vibratory Ejaculation

Naomi Betesh DO

Description

In males with SCI with ejaculatory dysfunction, electroejaculation and vibratory ejaculation are methods to induce ejaculation for sperm retrieval.

Key Principles

- Autonomic dysreflexia (AD) may occur in persons with injuries above T6 with either procedure.
- Detrusor contraction and retrograde ejaculation may occur with both methods.

Electroejaculation

- Electrical stimulation is given in a wavelike pattern of progressively increasing voltage until ejaculation occurs.
- Electroejaculation can be used on men with any type of SCI.

Penile vibratory stimulation

- Penile vibratory stimulation (PVS) requires an intact spinal cord at T11–S4 as this type of stimulation tries to activate the ejaculatory reflex.
- PVS is inexpensive, painless, and noninvasive.

Indications

- Males with ejaculatory dysfunction due to spinal cord disease or injury

Contraindications

- Inflammation of the glans penis
- Inability to understand directions
- Untreated hypertension
- Rectal lesions for electroejaculation

Special Considerations

- Electroejaculation can be painful if the individual has preserved sensation at or below the level of the abdomen; spinal or general anesthesia may be necessary.
- PVS must be applied with caution to a person with a penile prosthesis.
- Recently injured individuals may not respond to penile vibratory stimulation.

Key Procedural Steps

Electroejaculation

- The individual is catheterized to empty the bladder prior to the procedure (to prevent urine from adversely effecting any retrograde ejaculation).
- A sperm-friendly medium can be instilled into the bladder or the individual may take an oral alkalinating agent.
- Rectroscopy is performed prior to the procedure to make sure there are no rectal lesions.
- An electrical probe is placed in contact with the rectal wall near the prostate gland and seminal vesicles.
- A handheld vibrator is applied to the glans penis and the frenulum of the penis to trigger an ejaculatory reflex.
- Rhythmic electrical stimulation at progressively increasing voltages is given via the rectal probe.
- About 15 to 35 stimulations may be needed to produce adequate semen.
- When the procedure is finished, the bladder is catheterized to empty any retrograde ejaculation.
- Rectroscopy is repeated to make sure no injury occurred to the rectum from the procedure.

Penile vibratory stimulation

- The individual is positioned either sitting or supine.
- A vibrating disc is applied to the frenulum for 3 minutes or until ejaculation occurs.
- If after 3 minutes ejaculation does not occur, a rest period of 1 to 2 minutes is taken and then stimulation is repeated.

Anticipated Problems

- AD can occur in individuals with injuries above T6.
- Pretreat anyone with a history of AD.
- Individuals at risk for AD should have vital signs monitored during the procedure.
- Retrograde ejaculation may occur with either procedure but is more common with electroejaculation.
- Abdominal spasms, erections, or leg spasms may occur during penile vibratory stimulation.

■ Males with SCI may still be plagued with infertility even with successful ejaculation due to abnormal sperm motility and viability.

Helpful Hints

■ Sperm collection with PVS may be impaired in patients with a penile prosthesis.

Suggested Readings

Biering-Sorensen F, Sonksen J. Sexual function in spinal cord lesioned men. *Spinal Cord*. 2001;39:455–470.

Brackett NL, Nash MS, Lynne CM. Male fertility following spinal cord injury: facts and fiction. *Phys Ther*. 1996;76:1221–1231.

Brackett NL, Santa-Cruz C, Lynne CM. Sperm from spinal cord injured men lose motility faster than sperm from normal men: the effect is exacerbated at body compared to room temperature. *J Urol*. 1997;157:2150–2153.

Patki P, Woodhouse J, Hamid R, et al. Effects of spinal cord injury on semen parameters. *J Spinal Cord Med*. 2008;31(1):27–32.

Sønksen J, Ohl DA. Penile vibratory stimulation and electroejaculation in the treatment of ejaculatory dysfunction. *Int J Androl*. 2002;25(6):324–332.

Utida C, Truzzi JC, Bruschini H, et al. Male infertility in spinal cord trauma. *Int Braz J Urol*. 2005;31(4):375–383.

Sexuality and Reproduction: Labor and Delivery

Naomi Betesh DO

Description

Labor and delivery for individuals with SCI manifests with unique problems that need to be recognized and addressed. During delivery all women with lesions above T6 should be expected to experience autonomic dysreflexia (AD).

Key Principles

- Pain from the first stage of labor is transmitted via sympathetic fibers at T10–L1.
- Pain from the second stage of labor is due to distention of the perianal tissues via the pudendal nerve and the S2–S4 spinal segments.
- Women with cord transection above T10 may have painless labor.
- Women with SCI at lower segments may be unaware of uterine contractions.
- Labor may be perceived as back pain, increased spasticity, or AD.
- It is important to try to prevent unattended delivery in women with impaired ability to sense contractions.
- AD may occur during labor and delivery, even in women with no prior history of AD.
- Obstetrical staff must be educated regarding unique needs of individuals with SCI including pressure ulcer and injury prevention, signs, symptoms, and prevention of AD.

Special Considerations

- For women who are unable to be put into the lithotomy position due to spasticity or contracture, a side-lying position may be considered with the upper leg flexed at the hip.
- A contracted pelvis is more common in women with long-standing injury and may be an indication for cesarean section.
- In women with cervical lesions, pregnancy may further affect already impaired pulmonary function leading to the necessity for ventilatory support and respiratory care.
- Rate of preterm labor may be slightly increased after SCI.
- With increasing weight gain of pregnancy, self-transfers become more difficult.
- Muscle atrophy and osteoporosis secondary to SCI can contribute to pathologic fractures. Pregnant women should be transferred with care.
- Consider delivery in bed to avoid a transfer to delivery table.
- Women at risk for AD should deliver in a unit capable of invasive hemodynamic monitoring.
- In some women AD may be the only clinical manifestation of labor.

Key Procedural Steps

- In women with impaired uterine sensation, weekly cervical exams should begin at 28 weeks and hospital admission should occur once cervical dilation or effacement is noted.
- Individual should be repositioned every 2 hours during labor and delivery to prevent skin breakdown.
- Topical anesthetics should be used prior to urethral, bladder, rectal, vaginal/cervical manipulation.
- Body temperature should be monitored. However, temperature increases may be due to poor thermoregulation rather than intra-amniotic infections.
- Epidural or spinal anesthesia to T10 should be initiated early during labor to prevent AD.
- Continuous hemodynamic monitoring should be considered in any women at risk for AD.
- Appropriate short-acting, rapid onset antihypertensives should be readily available.
- Antihypertensives can be used if individual has AD prior to anesthesia initiation or in spite of anesthesia.
- If AD occurs during stage two of labor despite anesthesia, vaginal delivery can be expedited with forceps or vacuum.
- Cesarean section is indicated for intractable AD.

Anticipated Problems

- Episiotomy may precipitate AD.
- Hypotension, which is common in individuals with SCI, may be aggravated by hormonal decrease in systemic vascular resistance due to pregnancy.

Helpful Hints

- Refer pregnant individuals to anesthesiologist for antepartum evaluation with plan for epidural anesthesia at onset of labor.
- Uterine palpation should be reviewed with the pregnant individual to help her recognize labor.
- Symptoms that may indicate the onset of labor should be reviewed with the individual, including increased spasticity or abdominal or leg spasms.
- AD during labor tends to occur with contractions and resolves in between, whereas in pregnancy-induced hypertension the hypertension is constant.

Suggested Readings

ACOG Committee Opinion. Management of labor and delivery for patients with spinal cord injury. *Int J Gynecol Obstet.* 1991;36:253–254.

ACOG Committee Opinion. Obstetric management of patients with spinal cord injuries. *Int J Gynecol Obstet.* 2002;79:189–191.

Pereira, L. Obstetric management of the patient with spinal cord injury. *Obstet Gynecol Surv.* 2003;58(10):678–686.

Skin Management: Pressure Ulcers

Donald Macron MD MA

Description

Many factors contribute to the formation of pressure ulcers in persons with SCI. Management of pressure ulcers relies on pressure relief and maintenance of a beneficial wound healing environment.

Key Principles

- Pressure relief is the keystone of pressure ulcer prophylaxis and treatment.
- Pressure relief protocols (including positional changes and use of specialized support surfaces) are indicated in all individuals with sensorimotor impairment.
- When prevention fails, treatment involves keeping wounds clean, moist, and debrided.
- Necrosis and debris need to be cleared for optimal wound healing.
- Debridement removes a nidus for infection and a mechanical barrier to wound closure.
- Debridement of a wound permits accurate staging and depth assessment.
- Infected ulcers should be treated by mechanical and chemical means.
- Contributors to wound development should be identified and addressed.
- Clean wounds require protective, space-filling dressings.

Contraindications

- Dry eschar on the foot should be managed with pressure relief and protection, not debridement.
- Autolytic debridement (see below) is contraindicated in the setting of active surrounding infection.

Special Considerations

- Antiseptic or antimicrobial solutions should be used with care as some can harm fibroblasts and retard wound healing.
- Clinical judgment is needed to decide when debridement can be done at bedside, when surgical intervention is necessary, or when watchful waiting is appropriate.
- Cellulitis, sepsis, and osteomyelitis warrant intravenous antibiotics and prompt surgical consultation.

Key Procedural Steps

- Identify and relieve source of pressure.

Pressure relief

- Susceptible areas, such as bony prominences, should be given special attention in pressure relief protocols.
- Positional changes in bed should be performed every 2 hours.
- Seated weight shifts should be performed at least every 20 minutes for 2 minutes.
- Specialized support surfaces are used to distribute pressure away from pressure-sensitive areas.

Dressings

- Barrier dressings can be occlusive or semipermeable.
- Hydrocolloids, fillers, hydrogels, occlusive barrier films, and alginates promote autolytic debridement.
- Gauze dressings facilitate mechanical debridement.
- Vacuum-assisted closure (VAC) dressings can provide excellent results for healing deep or heavily draining ulcers.

Antibiotics and antiseptics

- Topical products can be considered for early erosions and local infections.
- Systemic antibiotics are appropriate for expanding areas of infection, sepsis or bacteremia, abscess or osteomyelitis.

Debridement

- Sharp debridement to remove necrotic tissue may be performed at bedside or in the operating room.
- Mechanical debridement uses mechanical means (wet-to-dry dressings, irrigation, dextranomers, whirlpool, etc.) to remove devitalized tissue and debris from a wound.
- Enzymatic debridement is a slower, more selective debridement using proteolytic enzymes to remove necrotic tissue, leaving granulation tissue unharmed.
- Autolytic debridement uses occlusive or semiocclusive wound dressings to facilitate endogenous enzymatic activity.

Modalities

- Modalities (such as diathermy, ultraviolet light, electrical stimulation, etc) can be considered as adjunctive therapy.

- Studies examining the efficacy of physical modalities in ulcer healing have been mixed.

Anticipated Problems

- Enzymatic debridement of large-area wounds is currently not cost-effective and impractical if used alone.
- Care must be taken with sharp debridement to avoid damage to vulnerable structures and viable tissue.
- Mechanical debridement is often very effective but can be time-consuming and labor-intensive, especially with contaminated wounds.
- Autolytic debridement should not be attempted with clear evidence of wound infection.
- Infection—notably osteomyelitis—can retard or prevent proper healing of pressure ulcers.

Helpful Hints

- Prevention of pressure ulcers and vigilant observation for recurrence is the mainstay of treatment.
- Proper positioning, pressure relief practices, and hygiene are all critical for wound prevention and resolution.

- All pressure ulcers should be considered colonized—not necessarily infected; wound cultures should be viewed skeptically in light of universal colonization.

Suggested Readings

Bluestein D, Javaheri A. Pressure ulcers: prevention, evaluation, and management. *Am Fam Phys.* 2008;78(10):1186–1194.

Consortium for Spinal Cord Medicine Clinical Practice Guidelines. Pressure ulcer prevention and treatment following spinal cord injury: a clinical practice guideline for health-care professionals. *J Spinal Cord Med.* 2001;24 (Suppl 1):S40–S101.

National Pressure Ulcer Advisory Panel. www.npuap.org

Rodeheaver GT. Pressure ulcer debridement and cleansing: a review of current literature. *Ostomy Wound Manage.* 1999;45(1A):80S–85S.

Romanelli M, Mastronicola D. The role of wound-bed preparation in managing chronic pressure ulcers. *J Wound Care.* 2002;11(8):305–310.

Thomas DR. Prevention and treatment of pressure ulcers: what works? what doesn't? *Cleve Clin J Med.* 2001;68(8):704–722.

Whitney J, et al. Guidelines for the treatment of pressure ulcers. *Wound Repair Regen.* 2006;14(6):663–679.

Section II: Interventions

Skin Management: Surgery for Pressure Ulcers

Donald Macron MD MA

Description

Myocutaneous flap repair is a reconstructive surgery used to treat advanced pressure ulcers after conservative measures fail.

Key Principles

- Procedure entails the transfer of a flap of healthy muscle and skin and blood supply to the area formerly occupied by the pressure lesion.
- Resultant reconstruction is approximately as resistant to future pressure ulcers as the original structures.
- A healed, intact flap provides a physiologic barrier to infection with return of full-thickness skin.
- Creation of the flap degrades or eliminates muscle function in the tissue used.
- Well-planned and well-constructed flaps significantly limit pressure, friction, and shearing damage at wound sites.

Indications

- Procedure is usually for stage III or IV sacral, ischial, or trochanteric ulcers unresponsive to conventional therapies.

Contraindications

- May be relatively contraindicated in ambulatory patients, as the potential loss of muscular function may outweigh the health benefits.
- Individuals who are unstable, have poor nutrition, or are unlikely to tolerate blood loss and general anesthesia are poor candidates for this procedure.

Special Considerations

- Location of the wound, level of motor function, and comorbidities all need consideration.
- Sometimes, the strategy of moving a sensate muscle to a region with sensory compromise may remind the patient to perform necessary pressure relief.

Key Procedural Steps

Preoperative

- Adequate debridement and infection control should be performed prior to surgery.
- Nutritional status should be optimized before surgery.
- Spasticity should be controlled to avoid stress on the repair.
- Bowels should be expurged before surgery to prevent soiling of the surgical site intraoperatively or postoperatively.
- Flap creation is usually preceded by the removal of the bursa and the wound's granulation base.

Intraoperative

- Judicious muscle selection and creation of a flap with a well-vascularized base increase the chances for healing success.
- Rotation, advancement, and free flaps are different techniques of filling in the tissue defect left by the ulcer excision.
- Excessive tension at the wound site can retard or prevent wound healing; allowances to minimize tension should be made during the surgery.
- Drains placed prior to wound closure minimize fluid accumulation beneath the flap.

Postoperative

- It is vital postoperatively to minimize sheering and tension across the surgical site.
- Pressure relief protocols need to be rigorously maintained.
- Postoperative care often requires several weeks of absolute pressure relief, with graduated return to sitting position, to preserve the flap integrity.

Anticipated Problems

- Statistically, it is common for myocutaneous flaps to develop ulceration recurrence, with estimates as high as 60%.
- Postoperative surveillance for wound dehiscence and necrosis is advised, as these are serious and not infrequent events.
- If the root causes of the original pressure ulcer are not addressed, any repair will be compromised by the same causes.
- Mechanical stress to the flap needs to be minimized postoperatively, as the repair is susceptible to tension and stress damage.

■ Lost sympathetic tone and impaired vasomotor response seen in many persons with SCI can result in the development of postoperative hematoma, potentially causing flap failure.

■ Spasticity needs to be monitored and controlled in the operative and postoperative periods if a flap is to have a chance of success.

Helpful Hints

■ Selection of transposed muscle depends on multiple factors—tissue viability, location of the wound, patient functional level, wound size, and so on—and is commonly taken from a variety of donor sites, including gracilis, tensor fascia lata, gluteus, hamstring, latissimus, sartorius, and trapezius.

Suggested Readings

Black JM, Black SB. Surgical management of pressure ulcers. *Nurs Clin North Am.* 1987;22(2):429–438.

Buntine JA, Johnstone B. The contributions of plastic surgery to care of the spinal cord injured patient. *Paraplegia.* 1988;26(2):87–93.

Consortium for Spinal Cord Medicine Clinical Practice Guidelines. Pressure ulcer prevention and treatment following spinal cord injury: a clinical practice guideline for health-care professionals. *J Spinal Cord Med.* 2001;24(Suppl 1):S40–S101.

Foster RD, Anthony JP, Mathes SJ, et al. Ischial pressure sore coverage: a rationale for flap selection. *Br J Plast Surg.* 1997;50:374–379.

Rubayi S, Cousins S, Valentine WA. Myocutaneous flaps. Surgical treatment of severe pressure ulcers. *AORN J.* 1990;52(1):40–45.

Sørensen JL, Jørgensen B, Gottrup F. Surgical treatment of pressure ulcers. *Am J Surg.* 2004;188(1A):42–51.

Skin Management: Wheelchair Seat Cushions and Bed Support Surfaces

Donald Macron MD MA

Description
Appropriate choice of mattress and wheelchair cushion is a crucial component of a comprehensive skin protection program.

Key Principles
- Pressure sores form when local tissue pressure exceeds capillary pressure, resulting in underperfusion and ischemia.
- Effective support distributes pressure broadly as possible to prevent high pressure at any point.
- Other strategies include automatic turning, and alternating pressure systems.

Indications
- Pressure-relieving mattresses and seating systems are indicated for all individuals with sensorimotor impairments.
- Degree of pressure relief needed depends on degree of impairment, risk factors for skin breakdown, and history of prior wounds.

Special Considerations
- The Braden and Gosnell Scales predict pressure ulcer risk and can also be used in selecting support surfaces.
- An individual's wound status and comorbidities also need consideration when choosing a surface.
- Regular repositioning is a mainstay of ulcer prevention with any support surface.
- Overlays that exhibit "bottoming out" with a specific individual should not be used.
- Donut or ring cushions can cause pressure ulcers, and should not be used.
- Head-of-bed elevation, especially past 25°, increases sacral shear forces and focal pressure.

Key Procedural Steps

Bed support surfaces
- Static supports such as foam overlays are appropriate for individuals with limited mobility who do not exhibit "bottoming out" or excess shear, and who can be repositioned on noncompromised tissue.
- Dynamic supports are reserved for individuals who cannot use static supports, particularly those with advanced ulcers or recent flap surgery.
- Foam overlays are inexpensive, low maintenance, versatile static supports, but have limited life and limited heat and moisture dissipation.
- Static flotation surfaces (air-, water-, gel-filled, etc) provide passive pressure reduction with pseudoimmersion, but need monitoring for over- and underfilling.
- Dynamic supports with alternating air-filled units provide intermittent pressure relief to the body and increasing blood flow (though no studies conclusively show this in practice).
- Low air-loss units are for individuals with multiple compromised surfaces who cannot tolerate regular positional changes; they provide excellent pressure reduction, heat and moisture control, and shear minimization.
- Air-fluidized (or high air-loss) units provide the most immersion and pressure distribution, and are chosen for individuals after myocutaneous flaps or with severe and widespread pressure ulceration.

Seat cushions
- Foam cushions (which can be flat or contoured) are inexpensive and low maintenance, but have a short lifespan and are susceptible to bottoming out.
- Gel- and fluid-filled cushions can mold to anatomical contours, may limit shearing, and provide improved pressure distribution.
- Air-filled cushions permit increased immersion and pressure distribution, but bottoming out, decreased stability and posture, and increased maintenance requirements (proper inflation and leakage) are added concerns.
- Air-filled cushions are also available as a matrix of multiple individual air-filled units, providing even better and more regional pressure relief.
- Dynamic air-filled units have been developed that sequentially inflate and deflate contiguous cells, much like alternating air-filled mattresses.

- Pressure mapping can be used as an adjunct in tailoring seat cushions and for indicating areas that may be at increased risk to pressure damage.

Anticipated Problems

- The cost of many specialized surfaces is substantial, and needs to be weighed against the risk of potential pressure ulcers to the individual.
- Air-, gel-, and fluid-filled surfaces often have to be filled and maintained in specific ranges to be effective.
- Maintenance of covers, underpads, proper cleaning and disinfecting are all important to optimize wound prevention and treatment; some surfaces are more labor-intensive in these regards than others.
- Air-fluidized beds have drying properties that (while usually beneficial or negligible) can aggravate respiratory or dehydration problems.

- Moisture and heat retention are issues with many impermeable surfaces.
- Independent bed mobility is significantly more difficult when using dynamic surfaces.

Suggested Readings

Clark M, Hiskett G, Russell L. Evidence-based practice and support surfaces: are we throwing the baby out with the bath water? *J Wound Care.* 2005;14(10): 455–458.

Garber SL, Dyerly LR. Wheelchair cushions for persons with spinal cord injury: an update. *Am J Occup Ther.* 1991;45(6):550–554.

Hess CT. Managing tissue loads. *Adv Skin Wound Care.* 2008;21(3):144.

McInnes E, Cullum NA, Bell-Syer SEM, et al. Support surfaces for pressure ulcer prevention. *Cochrane Database Syst Rev.* 2008;4(Art. No. CD001735).

Section II: Interventions

Spinal Decompression, Fusion, and Instrumentation

Youssef Josephson DO

Description

Surgical interventions used alone or in combination to relieve pressure or compression on the spinal cord and/or nerve roots or to stabilize an unstable spine.

Key Principles

Discectomy

- Removal of a portion of the entire intervertebral disc (IVD) to relieve pressure on the nerve roots or the spinal cord
- Microdiscectomy refers to removal of a small fragment of disc material preserving the remainder of the disc.

Laminotomy or laminectomy

- Involves removal of the lamina to increase the canal size and relieve pressure or to allow for placement of hardware

Corpectomy

- Removal of the vertebral body as well as the discs above and below

Spinal fusion

- Linking together of two or more adjacent vertebrae

Spinal instrumentation

- Placement of hardware on the spine to increase stability or to promote fusion

Indications

- Correction of deformity
- Stabilization of the spine
- Decompression of neural elements
- Vertebral fracture
- Spinal stenosis
- Infection
- Tumor
- Myelopathy with spinal cord compression
- Herniated nucleus pulposus

Contraindications

- Severe cardiac or pulmonary disease
- Advanced age with osteoporosis

Special Considerations

- Controversy exists on the timing and the benefit of "early" surgical intervention in traumatic SCI.
- Fehling et al. conducted a meta-analysis of the literature on early surgical intervention and found a significant benefit in animal models but that benefit was not reproduced in humans.
- The benefit in humans was most notable in incomplete lesions with obvious compression.

Key Procedural Steps

Discectomy

- The individual is placed in a prone position under general anesthesia.
- A small midline incision and careful exposure (clearing of posterior muscles) is performed.
- Laminectomy is usually performed.
- Disc material is removed.
- Cage or bone graft spacer can be placed to maintain disc height.

Microdiscectomy

- The individual is placed in a lateral decubitus position.
- An 18-gauge trocar is inserted 8 to 10 cm off midline at the desired level under fluoroscopic guidance.
- Once proper placement is confirmed by biplanar imaging, a cannula is inserted and a foot pedal controlled suction cutting device (Onik device) is introduced.
- When the disc fragment is removed, the remaining disc is then irrigated with antibiotic solution (bacitracin or gentamicin).

Laminectomy

- The individual is placed in a prone position under general anesthesia with monitoring.
- A midline incision is made and dissection is performed to reveal the desired spinal levels.
- Once the proper level is cleared, the lamina is removed laterally with an osteotome.
- Replacement of the lamina with a laminoplasty may be performed.

Corpectomy

- Either an anterior or posterior approach is selected based on injury.
- Exposure is obtained.
- Discectomy is performed above and below the corpectomy site to obtain visualization of the spinal canal.
- The annulus fibrosis is removed with a sharp knife.
- Vertebrectomy is completed with a high power drill.
- Allograft or autograft bone or a cage packed with fragments of the same is placed to maintain the disc height.
- Exposure for thoracic corpectomy requires thoracotomy and chest tube placement.

Fusion

- Various approaches exist and many different plate and screw options are available.
- Bone grafts are obtained prior to fusion.
- Once either discectomy, laminectomy, or corpectomy is performed, if the segment is deemed to be unstable screws are placed into the pedicles.
- Individuals are electrophysiologically monitored during instrumentation placement to monitor for possible injury.

Anticipated Problems

- Pain
- In the anterior cervical approaches, transient vocal cord paralysis, breathing problems, dysphagia, and odynophagia may occur.
- Worsening of neurologic injury
- Air embolus
- Brachial plexus injury
- Pseudoarthrosis
- Non healing of a fusion
- Infection
- Blood loss

Helpful Hints

- A clear understanding of a individual's injury is required for the surgeon to choose the proper surgical technique for good results to be obtained.

Suggested Readings

Fehlings M. The timing of surgical intervention in the treatment of spinal cord injury: a systemic review of recent clinical evidence. *Spine.* 2006;31(11)S28–S35.

Winn HR. *Youmans Neurological Surgery.* 1st ed. New York: Saunders; 2004.

Section II: Interventions

Spinal Orthoses

Donald Macron MD MA ■ Richard Freiden MD

Description
Spinal orthoses are used to restrict motion, provide support, facilitate fracture healing, and maintain spinal alignment.

Key Principles
- Devices vary as to motions restricted and portions of the spine controlled.
- Devices can be prefabricated or custom-made, and use a variety of metals, plastics, and foams.
- Instead of eponyms, modern device naming uses first-letter abbreviations of regions immobilized (eg, a TLSO is a thoracic-lumbar-sacral orthosis).
- Duration of use depends on stability of the region immobilized.

Indications
- There is a need to restrict vertebral movement in order to improve alignment, mechanically unload the spine, decrease pain, and/or to allow fracture and fusion healing.

Contraindications
- Avoid use if orthosis cannot provide sufficient stability or immobilization to the intended region.
- Avoid orthosis contact with open wounds and minimize pressure to vulnerable soft tissues.

Special Considerations
- Goals vary depending on injury location and severity, and surgical intervention.
- Orthosis selection and design depend upon device weight and size, cosmesis, comfort, ease of use and durability, and cost-effectiveness.
- Individuals with SCI often have limited respiratory reserve and are susceptible to visceral compression by some spinal orthoses.

Key Procedural Steps
- Selection should be based on the medical necessity for immobilization.
- Fit and alignment should be checked prior to orthosis customization, and again after the device has been used for at least 20 minutes.

- Must review device donning and doffing with both individual and caregivers.

Anticipated Problems
- Weak and atrophied muscles from prolonged immobilization
- Skin breakdown under the orthosis
- Orthosis migration and resultant discomfort
- Overheating and pooling of moisture under the orthosis
- Pin loosening, pin-site infections, and dural punctures with halo orthoses
- Impaired balance, stance, or gait of an otherwise functional individual due to an orthosis limiting the ability to make postural corrections and altering an individual's center of gravity

Helpful Hints

Cervical and cervical-thoracic orthoses
- Rigid collars (eg, Philadelphia, Aspen, Miami J) provide more stability than soft open-cell foam collars, and cover the region from the chin and occiput to the upper thorax.
- Poster appliances use vertical struts or "posters" to connect a base at the shoulders to an upper support at the mandible and occiput, further stabilizing cervical structures.
- A halo orthosis has a thoracic vest, a horizontal metal ring attached to the skull with pins, and several uprights connecting the two.
- The halo immobilizes the high cervical spine, and is used for Jefferson C1 fractures, unstable hangman's fractures, and odontoid fractures.
- Sternal-occipital-mandibular-immobilizer (SOMI) orthoses are used for C1 injuries, hangman's fractures, and provide good support from C4 rostrally.
- Minerva orthoses are rigid anterior posterior bivalved braces that support the neck and thoracic spine, and include a circumferential head strap attached to the posterior shell; they are used with C1 ring fractures and unstable hangman's fractures.
- The Yale brace is rigid cervical orthosis with a molded upper thoracic extension that immobilizes the low cervical region.

Thoracic, lumbar, and sacral orthoses

- A Raney Flexion lumbar sacral orthosis (LSO) provides pelvic encasement and abdominal compression, and allows some lumbar flexion.
- A Boston Overlap LSO is a rigid bivalve unit extending from the inferior scapular angle to the sacrococcygeal level and from the xiphoid to the pubis, which is used for stable mid- to low lumbar spinal lesions.
- LSOs and TLSOs are total contact orthoses that provide mid-thoracic and upper lumbar immobilization.

- A rigid hip joint/thigh cuff "spica" can increase support to the lower lumbar regions.

Suggested Readings

Giszter SF. Spinal cord injury: present and future therapeutic devices and prostheses. *Neurotherapeutics*. 2008;5(1):147–162.

Hsu JD, Michael JW, Fisk JR. *AAOS Atlas of Orthoses and Assistive Devices*. 4th ed. Boston: Elsevier Health Sciences; 2008.

Jaeger RJ, Yarkony GM, Roth EJ. Rehabilitation technology for standing and walking after spinal cord injury. *Am J Phys Med Rehabil*. 1989;68(3):128–133.

Sypert GW. External spinal orthotics. *Neurosurgery*. 1987;20(4):642–649.

Spinal Orthoses: Halo Placement and Management

Avniel Shetreat-Klein MD PhD

Description

A halo orthosis (or halo immobilization vest) minimizes motion of the cervical spine. It consists of a circumferential ring attached to the skull by means of four percutaneous pins. The ring is in turn attached to a thoracic vest by vertical uprights.

Key Principles

- The halo orthosis provides the most rigid immobilization for the cervical spine.
- The halo orthosis is particularly useful in stabilizing the C1–C2 segment.
- Application requires a knowledgeable practitioner to minimize risk of complications.
- Maintenance is more complicated as compared to other cervical orthoses, requiring, for example, daily pin care.

Indications

- Stabilization of high cervical spine after fracture or ligamentous injury (eg, Jefferson fractures, odontoid fractures, post-reduction stabilization of occipitocervical dislocation)
- May be used as preoperative immobilization, conservative nonoperative therapy, and as postoperative adjunct to internal fixation

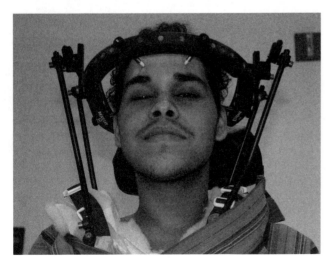

Halo orthosis.

- Has benefit of applying cervical traction, which other cervical orthoses cannot provide

Contraindications

- Osteoporosis
- Expected noncompliance with maintenance
- Cranial fractures
- Chest trauma
- Advanced age, respiratory compromise, and obesity are relative contraindications

Special Considerations

- No external device can provide 100% immobilization.
- Since immobilization in the halo vest is achieved by stabilizing relatively far above and below the c-spine, "snaking" or relative movement of the cervical vertebrae has been shown to occur, despite maintaining overall alignment of the c-spine as a whole.
- Modern halo devices are typically radiolucent and MRI safe.
- A wrench for emergency removal of the thoracic vest should be kept with the patient at all times.

Key Procedural Steps

- Local anesthetic, and possibly light sedation, is used for halo placement.
- A hard collar is kept in place for additional stability during halo placement.
- Sizing of the halo ring is based on measurement of the skull circumference at the cranial equator.
- The halo ring should be sized to be 1 to 2 inches from the skull at all points in the circumference.
- Anterior pins are situated in a "safe zone" located 1 cm superior to the orbital rim, at the lateral two-thirds of the orbit.
- Pins should be placed inferior to the greatest diameter of the skull to help prevent cephalad migration.
- Posterior pins are placed diagonally opposite to the anterior pins, just inferior to the greatest diameter of the skull.
- After appropriate local anesthesia, pins are placed directly through the skin, perpendicular to the skull surface.

- Pins are tightened with a torque wrench in 2 inch-pound increments, alternating pins diagonally, until an 8 inch-pound force is reached.
- Locknuts are then placed, with care not to overtighten.
- The posterior portion of the thoracic vest is placed and connected to the halo, followed by the anterior portion.
- Postapplication radiographs should be obtained.
- Pins should be retightened to an 8 inch-pound force at 48 hours.

Anticipated Problems
- Pin site infection
- Pin migration
- Pin loosening
- Pressure sore (under vest)
- Epidural abcess or dural tear from inadvertent cranial puncture
- Loss of reduction
- Respiratory compromise

Helpful Hints
- Pin sites should be cleaned daily with normal saline, Betadine, or hydrogen peroxide.
- Crusts should be gently removed.
- Lotions/creams are not needed and should be avoided.
- Infection is treated with oral antibiotics and local wound care.
- Nonresponse to antibiotics and local wound care is indication for pin removal and alternate placement.
- A loose pin may be retightened to an 8 inch-pound force only once.
- Subsequent reloosening is an indication for pin removal and alternate placement.

Suggested Readings
Botte MJ, Byrne TP, Abrams RA, Garfin SR. The halo skeletal fixator: current concepts of application and maintenance. *Orthopedics*. 1995;18(5):463–471.

Kang M, Vives MJ, Vaccaro AR. The halo vest: principles of application and management of complications. *J Spinal Cord Med*. 2003;26(3):186–192.

Tendon Transfers

Avniel Shetreat-Klein MD PhD

Description
The goal of so-called tendon transfer surgery for a person with SCI is to restore function at an impaired joint by surgically reassigning an intact muscle-tendon unit.

Key Principles
- The restoration of even a single functional movement such as key pinch can improve the quality of life and degree of independence of a person with tetraplegia.
- The International Classification for Surgery of the Hand in Tetraplegia systematically relates residual motor function to innervation.
- A successful tendon transfer requires a donor muscle that can demonstrate strong voluntary activation (≥4/5), and a recipient joint that has good passive ROM.
- It is preferable to choose a donor muscle that provides a redundant function, for example, transferring brachialis when biceps and brachioradialis will remain as functional elbow flexors.
- Nonredundant muscles can be chosen as donors when the function lost is not as crucial as the potential function gained.

Indications
- Tendon transfers are typically performed on those with C5–C7 neurologic levels of injury.
- Biceps to triceps or posterior deltoid to triceps tendon transfers can restore elbow extension.
- Active wrist extension can be generated with a brachialis to wrist extensor transfer.
- Key pinch and grip can be restored in someone with a C6 level injury with extensor carpi radialis to flexor digitorum profundus and brachioradialis to flexor pollicus longus transfers.

Contraindications
- Unwillingness or inability to undergo extensive postoperative hand therapy
- Joint contractures at recipient sites

Special Considerations
- Historically most authors recommend waiting 1 year postinjury before initiating surgery to allow for possible neurologic motor improvement.
- EMG is advisable to ascertain the degree of voluntary activation of a particular muscle.

- EMG is particularly important in instances where several potential donor muscles may be active for a given motion (eg, to assess whether the brachialis muscle is intact, EMG can verify that the clinically observed elbow flexion is not generated only by biceps or brachioradialis).
- Hand function is likely to have suboptimal function despite successful tendon transfer in a hand with little or no sensation.

Key Procedural Steps
- Specific surgical details depend on the particular donor and recipient sites involved.
- In general, donor muscle-tendon unit is dissected free of surrounding fascia.
- Tendon is left as long as possible to allow access to the recipient site without need for grafting.
- Maintaining intact nervous and vascular supply to the donor muscle is essential.
- Attention must be made to optimizing the donor muscle-tendon length to the available joint ROM to provide for the strongest muscle contraction after completion of healing.
- Intraoperative electrical stimulation can be performed to effectuate muscle contraction for assistance in tension setting.
- Various methods exist to attach donor tendon to the recipient site.
- Postoperative instructions for immobilization and eventual ROM vary by surgical procedure and surgeon preference.
- Typically there is a period of immobilization in a position that promotes maintenance of the appropriate tension, followed by progressive ROM and muscle re-education programs.

Anticipated Problems
- Wound infection
- Nerve injury
- Scar formation with loss of ROM
- Tendon rupture

Helpful Hints
- A recent survey of persons with tetraplegia indicated that 80% would undergo 2 to 3 months of decreased

independence after tendon transfer surgery if it would ultimately increase their function.

- Only 50% of persons with tetraplegia had heard of tendon transfer surgery.
- In a survey of postoperative individuals, 77% felt the surgery had a positive impact on their lives.

Suggested Readings

Anderson KD, Friden J, Lieber RL. Acceptable benefits and risks associated with surgically improving arm function in individuals living with cervical spinal cord injury. *Spinal Cord.* 2009;47:334–338.

Frost FM. Spinal cord injury medicine. In: Braddom R, ed. *Physical Medicine and Rehabilitation.* 2nd ed. Philadelphia: Saunders; 2000:1242–1243.

McDowell CL, Moberg EA, House JH. The second international conference on surgical rehabilitation of the upper limb in tetraplegia. *J Hand Surg Am.* 1986;11:604–608.

Wuolle KS, Bryden AM, Peckham PH, Murray PK, Keith M. Satisfaction with upper-extremity surgery in individuals with tetraplegia. *Arch Phys Med Rehabil.* 2003;84(8):1145–1149.

Wheelchair Prescription: Manual

Jenny Lieberman MSOTR/L ATP ■ Kristjan T. Ragnarsson MD

Description

The functional capabilities and postural alignment of a person with SCI are assessed in order to identify the optimal manual wheelchair design to facilitate mobility.

Key Principles

- Encourage independent mobility
- Facilitate function
- Halt the progression of deformity
- Promote good skin integrity

Indications

- Provide mobility for persons with SCI

Contraindications

- Upper extremity repetitive strain disorder (eg, tendonitis, carpal tunnel syndrome, epicondylitis, etc) or soft tissue damage (rotator cuff tear) are relative contraindications.
- Respiratory or cardiac insufficiency
- C1–C4 level of injury with an inability to propel independently

Special Considerations

- Skin integrity: existing pressure ulcer may necessitate special seating or positional change not ordinarily available in a manual wheelchair.
- Heterotopic ossification: decreased ROM at the hip and knee joints may require positioning that cannot be achieved in a manual wheelchair without negatively impacting alignment and skin integrity.
- Increased tone/spasticity: configuration of the frame design will have to be customized to decrease the onset of spasticity.
- Alignment: limitations in ROM can impact design of the frame and seating system.
- Function from the wheelchair: transfer technique and ability to complete self-care while seated can impact design of frame and seating system.
- Home accessibility: obstacles and doorway widths must be taken into consideration, when determining the wheelchair's frame dimensions.
- Transportability: how user will transport the wheelchair can determine the optimal shape of the frame and design of the seating system.

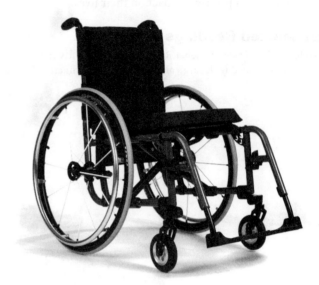

Ultra lightweight folding frame wheelchair.

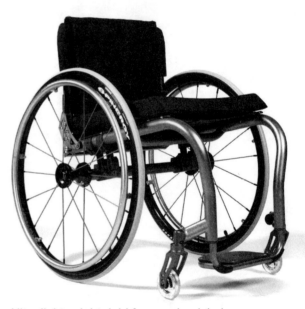

Ultra lightweight rigid frame wheelchair.

Key Procedural Steps

- Perform physical exam to assess muscle strength, sensation, ROM, bone and joint mobility, and integrity of the skin
- Perform individual detailed assessment of needs
- Set individual attainable goals with the user

- Provide a trial wheelchair and assess mobility, function, and alignment
- Generate an order with a vendor
- Complete a letter of medical necessity
- Facilitate delivery of wheelchair
- Train in use of wheelchair, including management and disassembly
- Adjust seating system and accessories as needed
- Provide follow-up by allowing the user to return for repairs and updating of wheelchair as needed

Anticipated Problems
- Insufficient insurance benefits
- Poor maintenance of equipment

- Need to modify rear wheel location for mobility skills

Helpful Hints
- The user should be an active participant in the entire process for the goals to be met and to prevent abandonment of equipment.

Suggested Reading
Paralyzed Veterans of America Consortium for Spinal Cord Medicine. Preservation of upper limb function following spinal cord injury: a clinical practice guideline for health care professionals. *J Spinal Cord Med.* 2005;28(5):434–470.

Section II: Interventions

Wheelchair Prescription: Power

Jenny Lieberman MSOTR/L ATP ■ Kristjan T. Ragnarsson MD

Description
The functional capabilities and postural alignment of a person with SCI with impaired upper extremity motor function, postural deformity, respiratory compromise, or impairment in skin integrity are assessed in order to identify the optimal power wheelchair design to facilitate independent mobility.

Key Principles
■ Encourage independent mobility
■ Facilitate function
■ Halt the progression of deformity
■ Promote good skin integrity

Indications
■ For persons with SCI who cannot walk or independently propel a manual wheelchair
■ Upper limb repetitive strain disorder and soft tissue damage that precludes use of a manual wheelchair
■ Respiratory or cardiac insufficiency that precludes use of a manual wheelchair
■ Significant impairment in skin integrity and an inability to shift weight in the seated position

Contraindications
■ Ability to independently maneuver in a manual wheelchair in all environments and complete all mobility-related activities of daily living (toileting, feeding, dressing, grooming, and bathing)
■ Significant cognitive or perceptual impairment rendering power mobility unsafe

Special Considerations
■ Skin integrity: Existing pressure ulcer may necessitate the addition of power seat functions to facilitate positional change for wound healing and skin protection.
■ Increased tone/spasticity may require special positioning; though, some power seat functions can trigger the onset of spasticity (eg, power recline and power elevating leg rests).
■ Alignment: Limitations in ROM (due to heterotopic ossification, deformity, or poor joint integrity) may require the addition of power seat functions for proper positioning and to increase function.

■ Function from the wheelchair: transfer technique and ability to complete self-care while seated can influence design of frame and seating system.
■ Home accessibility: Obstacles, including stairs and doorway widths, must be taken into consideration when considering powered mobility.
■ Users with impaired cognition may require special customization of the electronics to simplify control. Powered mobility may be contraindicated if unsafe operation is likely.
■ Users with impairment in perception or vision may require special customization of electronics or wheelchair controls to use alternative sensory pathways for feedback. Powered mobility may be contraindicated if affecting safety.

Key Procedural Steps
■ Perform history and physical exam to assess physical condition, including neurologic, musculoskeletal, skin, and cardiopulmonary function
■ Set attainable goals with the user
■ Provide a trial wheelchair to assess mobility, function, and alignment
■ Generate an order with a vendor
■ Complete a letter of medical necessity
■ For users with Medicare insurance, additional documentation is required. Specifically, face-to-face medical evaluation, prescription for mobility device, and a detailed written order.
  – The face-to-face medical evaluation consists of an office visit note (or medical chart note while in an inpatient facility) identifying why the user cannot walk, propel a manual wheelchair, or control a scooter within the home. Of greatest importance is the statement that a face-to-face visit took place. The note must indicate cognitive capabilities and address user motivation.
  – The documented date for the completion of the face-to-face evaluation: If a licensed/certified medical professional (LCMP), such as an occupational or physical therapist, is involved in the assessment, this is the date the physician signed the letter of medical necessity.
  – Facilitate delivery of wheelchair
  – Train in use of wheelchair, including management of electronics, seating system, and accessories

– Adjust electronics, seating system, and accessories as needed
– Provide follow-up by allowing the user to return for repairs and updating of wheelchair as needed

Anticipated Problems

■ Insufficient insurance benefits
■ Poor maintenance of equipment

Helpful Hints

■ The user should be an active participant in the entire process for the goals to be met and to prevent abandonment of equipment.
■ Conference with other professionals involved in patients care (eg, when there is impaired cognition and/or visual perception).

Suggested Readings

Local Coverage Decision (LCD) for Power Mobility Devices (L21271). CMS pub. 100–3, *Medicare National Coverage Determination Manual*. Chapter 1, Section 280.3.

Rehabilitation Engineering and Assistive Technology Society of North America. *RESNA Position on the Application of Seat-Elevating Devices for Wheelchair Users*. Arlington: RESNA; 2005.

Rehabilitation Engineering and Assistive Technology Society of North America. *RESNA Position on the Application of Tilt, Recline and Elevating Legrests for Wheelchair Users*. Arlington: RESNA; 2008.

Rehabilitation Engineering and Assistive Technology Society of North America. *RESNA Position on the Application of Wheelchair Standing Devices (2007)*. Arlington: RESNA; 2005.

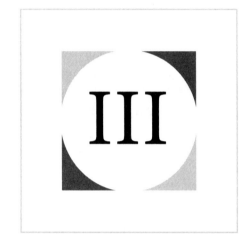

Outcomes

Wheelchair Skills: Manual

Liron Bensimon DPT CSCS ▧ Kristjan T. Ragnarsson MD

Description
Manual wheelchair mobility skills include propulsion, falling, and negotiation of ramps, curbs, and stairs.

Key Principles
- Propulsion effectiveness is dependent on the wheelchair weight, design, and the match between the seat and the user's body dimensions.
- Ride and seating comfort is dependent on the design and composition of the frame, seat, cushion, and tires, as well as the wheel and frame stiffness.

Indications
- Inability to ambulate safely and efficiently
- Need for household and/or community mobility

Contraindications
- Upper limb impairment prohibiting propulsion
- Cognitive deficits interfering with safe wheelchair mobility

Special Considerations
- Learning to do a wheelie is essential for managing uneven surfaces, ascending/descending ramps, and curbs, preventing front casters from becoming stuck.

Key Procedural Steps

Propel wheelchair
- Use long smooth propulsion strokes to limit hand and wrist impact on the pushrim and to minimize stroke frequency.
- A stroke pattern where the hand traces a semicircular pattern is the most efficient and least stressful on upper limbs.

Fall backwards in wheelchair safely
- Tuck in chin
- Place one arm behind head
- Use other arm to prevent knees from flexing into body

Ascend a ramp
- Lean forward as much as possible
- Use short quick arm strokes to maintain forward momentum

Descend a ramp
- Lean backwards as much as possible
- Allow pushrims to smoothly glide through the hands
- Grasp pushrim to slow down
- If grasp is weak, push medially on hand rims
- On steep ramps use a wheelie to keep from falling out of chair or follow a zig-zag path

Ascend a curb
- Approach curb in a forward direction
- Perform a wheelie to place casters up on curb
- Lean forward and firmly propel rear wheels onto curb

Descend a curb backwards
- Approach curb backward to the edge
- Lean forward and slowly propel backwards to lower rear wheels down
- Making a sharp turn to lower caster wheels down

Descend a curb forward
- Approach curb forward in a wheelie position
- Slowly lower rear wheels down curb

Ascend stairs alone
- Approach stairs backwards
- Tilt wheelchair back against first step
- Use one hand to pull handrail while other hand pulls on handrail or pushrim
- Reposition hands for next step and repeat

Descend stairs alone backwards
- Approach first step cautiously backwards
- Lean forward in chair
- Use both hands on handrail *or* one hand on handrail and other hand on pushrim
- Lower rear wheels down steps

Descend stairs alone forward
- Approach stairs forward in a wheelie position
- Maintain hands on pushrim to hold wheelie position
- Lower rear wheels down steps

Ascend and descend stairs with assistance
- The first assistant stands behind the wheelchair and pulls on the push handles with the wheelchair in a wheelie position.
- The second assistant stands in front of the wheelchair and ensures that the chair does not roll forward.

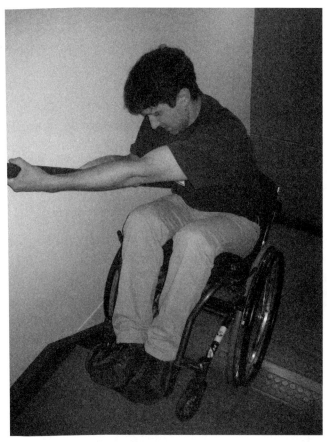

Descending stairs backwards.

Ascend and descend on buttocks
- Transfer from wheelchair onto the floor
- Bump up or down each step on buttocks
- Pull wheelchair to step beside buttocks after each step

Anticipated Problems
- Shoulder pain due to arthritis and rotator cuff tendonopathy
- Wrist and hand pain due to repetitive contact neuropathy
- Thumb pain due to arthritis

Helpful Hints
- A power-assist wheelchair can diminish repetitive stress on joints and nerves
- Obtain the lightest possible wheelchair that can meet the user's needs
- Use antitippers on wheelchair until comfortable performing wheelies
- Start with small obstacles and gradually increase the size of the obstacles

Suggested Reading
Koontz A, Shea M. Wheelchair skills. In: Sisto SA, Druin E, Sliwinski MM, et al., eds. *Spinal Cord Injuries Management and Rehabilitation*. St. Louis: Mosby; 2008:351–379.

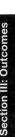

Section III: Outcomes

C1 to C3 Tetraplegia

Gina Armstrong MD ▪ Naomi Betesh DO ▪ Thomas N. Bryce MD

Key Innervated Muscles
- Cervical paraspinals
- Neck accessory muscles
- Sternocleidomastoid
- Trapezius
- Diaphragm partially innervated at C3 level

Available Muscle Actions
- Neck flexion, extension, rotation

Functional Outcomes

Medical
- Ventilator or phrenic/diaphragm-pacer–dependent, or may be able to breathe on own (C3).
- Total assistance may be needed to clear secretions with chest percussion and assistive coughs due to weak cough and low vital capacity.
- Appropriate bladder management options include continuous drainage with an indwelling suprapubic, transurethral catheter, or, for men only, reflex voiding with condom catheter drainage.
- Total assistance needed for inserting indwelling urinary catheter or applying external condom catheter and emptying urinary drainage bag.
- Appropriate bowel management includes a daily or every other day routine on a recliner commode or in bed.
- Total assistance needed for performance of bowel routine with digital stimulation and insertion of suppository or mini enema.

Activities of daily living
- Independent for pressure reliefs with a tilt-in-space power wheelchair with head or sip-and-puff controls
- Total assistance needed for dressing, eating, bathing, grooming, and brushing teeth
- Independent to total assist needed for communication and telephoning, depending on adaptive devices such as a mouth stick and high-tech computer
- Total assistance needed for all housework and kitchen work

Mobility
- Total assistance needed for transportation in an accessible van or public transportation
- Total assistance needed for bed mobility

- Total assistance needed for wheelchair and bed transfers. Independent in directing all transfers including hydraulic lift transfer
- Independent with power wheelchair propulsion with an appropriate control device such as a sip and puff control or head array
- Total assistance needed for manual wheelchair propulsion

Vocational
- 14% of persons with C1–C4 tetraplegia are employed.
- 65% work >30 hours per week.
- Of those with less than high school education, 1.4% are employed.
- Of those with high school education, 8% are employed.
- Of those with a bachelor's degree, 36% are employed.
- Of those with master's or doctoral degree, 61% are employed.
- Telework is an emerging way to return to the workforce.
- With Internet access and the use of a special mouse controlled by head movements, persons with high tetraplegia can overcome barriers to returning to work.

Participation in sports
- Individuals with high tetraplegia can participate in air rifle competitions.
- Assistance is allowed for loading, unloading, cocking the gun, and exchanging the target.
- A sip-and-puff device is then used to activate the trigger.

Prognosis

Motor recovery
- Most upper extremity recovery occurs during the first 6 months.
- Individuals without sacral sensory sparing of pinprick or residual motor function in any limb at 1 month are unlikely to regain any motor function in any limb.

Life expectancy
- A nonventilator-dependent 25-year-old can expect to live 33 years.
- A ventilator-dependent 25-year-old can expect to live 15 to 20 years.

- A nonventilator-dependent 50-year-old can expect to live 14 years.
- A ventilator-dependent 50-year-old can expect to live 5½ years.
- A nonventilator-dependent 75-year-old can expect to live 2½ years.
- A ventilator-dependent 75-year-old can expect to live <6 months.

Helpful Hints

- Caregivers need to be trained in proper body mechanics for transfers, dressing, and bathing individual.
- 94% of ventilator-independent persons with C1–C4 tetraplegia and at least 88% of ventilator-assisted persons note that they are glad to be alive when asked.

Suggested Readings

Apple D. *Physical Fitness: A Guide for Individuals with Spinal Cord Injury.* Baltimore: Department of Veterans Affairs; 1996.

Consortium for Spinal Cord Medicine. Outcomes following traumatic spinal cord injury: clinical practice guidelines for health-care professionals. *J Spinal Cord Med.* 2000;23(4):289–316.

Fisher CG, Noonan VK, Smith DE, et al. Motor recovery, functional status, and health-related quality of life in patients with complete spinal cord injuries. *Spine.* 2005;30(19):2200–2207.

National Spinal Cord Injury Statistical Center, University of Alabama at Birmingham. *2006 Annual Statistical Report.* July 2006.

Sisto SA, Durin E, Sliwinski MM. *Spinal Cord Injuries Management and Rehabilitation.* 1st ed. Missouri: Mosby; 2009.

C4 Tetraplegia

Gina Armstrong MD ■ Naomi Betesh DO ■ Thomas N. Bryce MD

Key Innervated Muscles
- All muscles innervated by C3
- Diaphragm
- Infraspinatus
- Levator scapulae

Available Muscle Actions
- Neck flexion, extension, rotation
- Scapula elevation
- Inspiration

Functional Outcomes

Medical
- May breathe on their own or be ventilator or phrenic/diaphragm-pacer–dependent; however, most are able to be weaned off the ventilator
- Total assistance may be needed to clear secretions with chest percussion and assistive coughs due to weak cough and low vital capacity.
- Appropriate bladder management options include continuous drainage with an indwelling suprapubic or transurethral catheter or for men only reflex voiding with condom catheter drainage.
- Total assistance needed for inserting indwelling urinary catheter or applying external condom catheter and emptying urinary drainage bag
- Appropriate bowel management includes a daily or every other day routine on a recliner commode or in bed.
- Total assistance needed for performance of bowel routine with digital stimulation and insertion of suppository or mini enema

Activities of daily living
- Independent for pressure reliefs with a tilt-in-space power wheelchair with head, pneumatic or sip-and-puff controls
- Total assistance needed for dressing, eating, bathing, grooming, and teeth brushing
- However, individuals with C4 tetraplegia with some elbow flexion and deltoid strength may use a mobile arm support to assist with feeding, grooming, and bathing
- Independent to total assist needed for communication and telephoning, depending on adaptive devices

- Telephoning can be achieved independently with speakerphone and mouthstick used to dial, or with voice recognition
- A mouthstick can be used for typing on the computer or with an implement holder and pencil or pen for writing
- Voice recognition systems can be used for the computer
- Total assistance needed for all housework and kitchen work

Mobility
- Total assistance needed for transportation in an accessible van or public transportation
- Total assistance needed for bed mobility
- Total assistance needed for wheelchair and bed transfers
- Independent in directing all transfers, including hydraulic lift transfer
- Independent with power wheelchair propulsion with an appropriate control device such as a sip-and-puff control or head array
- Total assistance needed for manual wheelchair propulsion

Vocational
- Individuals returning to work are more likely to start a new job than to return to their previous employment.
- One year postinjury, 14% of persons with tetraplegia were working.
- 5% of spinal cord-injured individuals work in a professional specialty 5 years postinjury.

Participation in sports
- Individuals with C4 tetraplegia can play chess using a computer with voice-activated software to verbalize which chess piece to advance and the computer will move the piece on the computer screen for them.

Prognosis

Motor recovery
- Most upper extremity recovery occurs during the first 6 months.
- Individuals with 1/5 or 2/5 muscle strength in the elbow flexors 1 month after injury will likely progress

to 3/5 or greater muscle strength in the elbow flexors by 1 year.

Life expectancy

- A 25-year-old can expect to live 32 years, in contrast to the normal life expectancy of 54 years.
- A 50-year-old can expect to live 13 years, in contrast to the normal life expectancy of 31 years.
- A 75-year-old can expect to live 2½ years, in contrast to the normal life expectancy of 12 years.

Helpful Hints

- Caregivers need to be trained in proper body mechanics for transfers, dressing, and bathing individual.
- 30% of ventilator-independent persons with C1–C4 tetraplegia report an excellent quality of life (QOL).
- 50% report a good QOL.

- 5% report a poor QOL, and the remainder report an average QOL.

Suggested Readings

Consortium for Spinal Cord Medicine. Outcomes following traumatic spinal cord injury: clinical practice guidelines for health-care professionals. *J Spinal Cord Med.* 2000; 23(4):289–316.

Fisher CG, Noonan VK, Smith DE, et al. Motor recovery, functional status, and health-related quality of life in patients with complete spinal cord injuries. *Spine.* 2005;30(19):2200–2207.

Hall KM, Knudsen ST, Wright J, Charlifue SW, Graves DE, Werner P. Follow-up study of individuals with high tetraplegia (C1–C4) 14 to 24 years postinjury. *Arch Phys Med Rehabil.* 1999;80(11):1507–1513.

National Spinal Cord Injury Statistical Center, University of Alabama at Birmingham. *2006 Annual Statistical Report.* July 2006.

Section III: Outcomes

C5 Tetraplegia

Gina Armstrong MD ▪ Naomi Betesh DO ▪ Thomas N. Bryce MD

Key Innervated Muscles

- All C1–C4 innervated muscles
- Deltoid
- Biceps
- Brachialis
- Brachioradialis
- Rhomboid
- Serratus anterior

Available Muscle Actions

- Elbow flexion and supination
- Shoulder flexion/abduction/extension
- Scapular abduction/adduction
- Neck flexion, extension, rotation
- Scapula elevation
- Inspiration

Functional Outcomes

Medical

- Total assistance may be needed to clear secretions with chest percussion and assistive coughs due to weak cough and low vital capacity.
- Appropriate bladder management options include continuous drainage with an indwelling suprapubic or transurethral catheter or for men-only reflex voiding with condom catheter drainage.
- Total assistance needed for inserting indwelling urinary catheter or applying external condom catheter and emptying urinary drainage bag.
- Appropriate bowel management includes a daily or every other day routine on a recliner commode or in bed.
- Total assistance needed for performance of bowel routine with digital stimulation and insertion of suppository or mini enema.

Activities of daily living

- Independent for pressure reliefs with a tilt-in-space power wheelchair with hand controls
- Total assistance needed for upper and lower body dressing
- Minimum assistance and set up needed for teeth brushing and grooming with adaptive equipment such as a wrist support with a utensil holder
- Total assistance needed for set up of meals, which includes cutting the food into bite-sized pieces

- Independent in feeding with adaptive equipment such as a wrist splint with utensil holder or universal cuff, bent fork or spoon, nonslip mat, plate guard, and possibly a mobile arm support
- Independent to some assistance after setup for communication with adaptive devices such as mobile arm support and universal cuff with pocket
- Telephoning may require a universal cuff to hold the eraser end of a pencil for dialing or a Bluetooth type device
- Total assistance needed for all housework and kitchen work

Mobility

- Independent driving a van with wheelchair lift and hand controls from secured wheelchair
- Moderate to maximum assistance needed for bed mobility
- Maximal assistance needed for sliding board transfers. Independent in directing all transfers, including hydraulic lift transfer
- Independent with power wheelchair propulsion with an arm-drive control
- Independent with manual wheelchair with modified hand rims indoors

Vocational

- 14% of persons with C5–C8 tetraplegia are employed.
- 66% work >30 hours per week.
- Of those with more than high school education, 3% are employed.
- Of those with master's and doctoral degrees, 62% are employed.

Participation in sports

- Individuals can participate in archery with assistance in putting the arrow on the bow, and with drawing and releasing the arrow.
- There is an adapted hook device that attaches to the palm of the hand that allows the archer to pull the bow with the use of the deltoid and biceps.

Prognosis

Motor recovery

- Most upper extremity recovery occurs during the first 6 months.

- 95% of individuals with 1/5 or 2/5 wrist extensor strength at 1 month will recover 3/5 strength in the wrist extensors by 1 year.

Life expectancy

- A 25-year-old can expect to live 36 years, in contrast to the normal life expectancy of 54 years.
- A 50-year-old can expect to live 16 to 20 years, in contrast to the normal life expectancy of 31 years.
- A 75-year-old can expect to live 4 to 6 years, in contrast to the normal life expectancy of 12 years.

Helpful Hints

- Sitting in an upright position helps the patient to use other gravity-assisted muscles to substitute for triceps.

- Wrist splints are needed to help maintain wrists in a neutral position during functional activities.

Suggested Readings

Consortium for Spinal Cord Medicine. Outcomes following traumatic spinal cord injury: clinical practice guidelines for health-care professionals. *J Spinal Cord Med.* 2000;23(4):289–316.

Fisher CG, Noonan VK, Smith DE, et al. Motor recovery, functional status, and health-related quality of life in patients with complete spinal cord injuries. *Spine.* 2005;30(19):2200–2207.

Krause JS, Kewman D, DeVivo MJ, et al. Employment after spinal cord injury: an analysis of cases from the model spinal cord injury systems. *Arch Phys Med Rehabil.* 1999;80(11):1492–1500.

National Spinal Cord Injury Statistical Center, University of Alabama at Birmingham. *2006 Annual Statistical Report.* July 2006.

Section III: Outcomes

C6 Tetraplegia

Gina Armstrong MD ■ Naomi Betesh DO ■ Thomas N. Bryce MD

Key Innervated Muscles
- All C1–C5 innervated muscles
- Clavicular pectoralis
- Serratus anterior
- Latissimus dorsi
- Supinator
- Extensor carpi radialis longus and brevis

Available Muscle Actions
- Elbow flexion and supination
- Shoulder flexion/abduction/extension
- Scapular abduction/adduction/protraction/elevation
- Neck flexion, extension, rotation
- Tenodesis causing thumb and index finger opposition with flexion
- Some horizontal adduction
- Forearm supination
- Radial wrist extension

Functional Outcomes

Medical
- Assistance may be needed to clear secretions if respiratory infection present.
- Continuous drainage with a catheter is the most common bladder management option for women with C6 level of injury and assistance is needed for inserting transurethral catheters.
- A continent urinary diversion (Mitrofanoff procedure) with an abdominal stoma placed for bladder access can allow a woman to catheterize herself independently.
- For men continuous catheter drainage, intermittent catheterization, or reflex voiding with condom catheter drainage are appropriate options.
- Men can be independent with intermittent catheterization or inserting indwelling urinary catheters using assistive devices.
- Assistance is usually needed for applying external condom catheters.
- Appropriate bowel management includes a daily or every other day routine on a recliner commode or in bed.
- Modified independence for actual performance of the invasive portion of bowel routine with rectal stimulation using an adapted tool and insertion of a suppository using a suppository inserter with mirror guidance on a commode.
- Assistance needed for setup and cleanup after bowel routine

Activities of daily living
- Independent for pressure reliefs in a manual or power wheelchair
- Modified independence with upper body dressing with button and zipper aids
- Some to total assistance needed for lower body dressing with adaptive devices, for example, loops on pants and socks, and Velcro on shoes
- Independent for toothbrushing with a universal cuff or electric toothbrush
- Independent with upper extremity bathing and some to total assistance needed with lower body bathing with adaptive equipment, for example, a wash mitt, handheld shower, lever-type faucet, grab bars, and roll in shower chair
- Independent in eating with or without adaptive equipment such as a utensil holder or universal cuff, bent fork or spoon, nonslip mat, plate guard
- Cutting food requires total assistance
- Independent to some assistance after setup for communication with or without adaptive devices such as a typing splint
- Total assistance needed for all housework and kitchen work

Mobility
- Independent driving a van with wheelchair lift and hand controls from secured wheelchair
- Minimum assistance to independent for bed mobility
- Minimal assistance to modified independent with transfer board for transfers on even surfaces
- Uneven surface transfers usually require assistance
- Independent with power wheelchair propulsion with standard arm controls
- Independent with manual wheelchair indoors

Vocational
- 23% of persons with C5–C8 tetraplegia are employed.

Participation in sports
- Quad rugby, developed in the 1970s, is a mix of basketball, ice hockey, and football. It is played on a

basketball court with a volleyball. A goal is scored when a player crosses the opponent's goal line while in possession of the ball.

Prognosis

Motor recovery

■ Most upper extremity recovery occurs during the first 6 months.
■ 95% of individuals with 1/5 or 2/5 finger or elbow extensor strength at 1 month will recover 3/5 strength in those extensors by 1 year.

Life expectancy

■ A 25-year-old can expect to live 36 years, in contrast to the normal life expectancy of 54 years.
■ A 50-year-old can expect to live 16 to 20 years, in contrast to the normal life expectancy of 31 years.

■ A 75-year-old can expect to live 4 to 6 years, in contrast to the normal life expectancy of 12 years.

Helpful Hints

■ Limit stretching of finger flexor and thumb adductor tendons in order to facilitate tenodesis grasp

Suggested Readings

Consortium for Spinal Cord Medicine. Outcomes following traumatic spinal cord injury: clinical practice guidelines for health-care professionals. *J Spinal Cord Med.* 2000;23(4):289–316.

Fisher CG, Noonan VK, Smith DE, et al. Motor recovery, functional status, and health-related quality of life in patients with complete spinal cord injuries. *Spine.* 2005;30(19):2200–2207.

National Spinal Cord Injury Statistical Center, University of Alabama at Birmingham. *2006 Annual Statistical Report.* July 2006.

C7 Tetraplegia

Gina Armstrong MD ■ Naomi Betesh DO ■ Thomas N. Bryce MD

Key Innervated Muscles
- All C1–C6 innervated muscles
- Triceps
- Sternal pectoralis
- Latissimus dorsi
- Extensor carpi radialis
- Flexor carpi radialis

Partially innervated:
- Extensor carpi ulnaris
- Extensor digitorum
- Extensor pollicis
- Extensor indicis
- Abductor pollicis longus

Available Muscle Actions
- All shoulder, neck, and scapular movements
- Elbow flexion and extension
- Ulnar wrist extension
- Some finger extension
- Some thumb abduction
- Forearm supination
- Radial wrist extension and flexion

Functional Outcomes

Medical
- Assistance may be needed to clear secretions in the setting of severe respiratory infection.
- For men, continuous suprapubic catheter drainage, intermittent catheterization, or reflex voiding with condom catheter drainage are appropriate bladder management options.
- Men can be independent with intermittent catheterization using assistive devices.
- For women, independent self-catheterization is possible, but it is technically difficult and time consuming and is generally not practical.
- Other options for women include continuous drainage with a transurethral catheter or a continent urinary diversion with an abdominal stoma.
- Women may be independent or may need assistance for emptying a urinary drainage bag.
- Appropriate bowel management includes a daily or every other day routine on a padded commode.
- Potentially independent for performance of bowel routine with assistive devices including a digital stimulator, suppository inserter, and mirror.

Activities of daily living
- Independent pressure reliefs
- Modified independent upper and lower body dressing with adaptive equipment such as button and zipper aids
- Modified independent teeth cleaning with built up toothbrush, electric toothbrush, or universal cuff
- Independent upper extremity bathing and some to total assistance needed with lower body bathing with adaptive equipment, for example, a wash mitt, hand-held shower, lever-type faucet, grab bars, and tub transfer bench or preferably a roll-in shower chair
- Independent eating after setup although may need universal cuff or utensils with built up handles
- Independent to some assistance after setup for use of telephone and writing
- A typing splint is often necessary for typing
- Independent light meal preparation and light housework
- Total assistance needed for heavy housework

Mobility
- Independent driving a car or van with hand controls
- Minimum assistance to independent for bed mobility
- Minimal assistance to modified independent with transfer board for transfers
- Independent power wheelchair mobility
- Independent ultra lightweight manual wheelchair mobility with modified hand rims

Vocational
- Three-fourths of those with a C7 level of injury are unemployed.
- Two-thirds of those with a C7 level of injury who are working work >30 hours per week.

Participation in sports
- Individuals can participate in track races with distances from 1,000 meters through marathons.
- Specialized racing wheelchairs are used that are customized for each individual.

Prognosis

Motor recovery

- Most upper extremity recovery occurs during the first 6 months post-injury.

Life expectancy

- A 25-year-old can expect to live 36 years, in contrast to the normal life expectancy of 54 years.
- A 50-year-old can expect to live 16 to 20 years, in contrast to the normal life expectancy of 31 years.
- A 75-year-old can expect to live 4 to 6 years, in contrast to the normal life expectancy of 12 years.

Helpful Hints

- Minimize the number of transfers per day to prevent upper extremity overuse.
- Whenever possible encourage your patients to grip the edge of the surface they are transferring to prevent carpal tunnel syndrome.

Suggested Readings

Consortium for Spinal Cord Medicine. Outcomes following traumatic spinal cord injury: clinical practice guidelines for health-care professionals. *J Spinal Cord Med.* 2000;23(4):289–316.

Fisher CG, Noonan VK, Smith DE, et al. Motor recovery, functional status, and health-related quality of life in patients with complete spinal cord injuries. *Spine.* 2005;30(19):2200–2207.

Krause JS, Kewman D, DeVivo MJ, et al. Employment after spinal cord injury: an analysis of cases from the model spinal cord injury systems. *Arch Phys Med Rehabil.* 1999;80(11):1492–1500.

National Spinal Cord Injury Statistical Center, University of Alabama at Birmingham. *2006 Annual Statistical Report.* July 2006.

C8 Tetraplegia

Gina Armstrong MD ■ Naomi Betesh DO ■ Thomas N. Bryce MD

Key Innervated Muscles
- All C1–C7 innervated muscles
- Flexor digitorum profundus and superficialis
- Abductor pollicis longus

Partially innervated:
- Lumbricals
- Abductor pollicis brevis
- Opponens pollicis
- Flexor pollicis brevis
- Adductor pollicis
- Palmar brevis
- Abductor digiti minimi
- Flexor digiti minimi
- Opponens pollicis
- Interossei

Available Muscle Actions
- All movements of neck, shoulders, scapulas, elbows
- Wrist flexion/extension
- Finger flexion/extension
- Thumb abduction/flexion/extension

Functional Outcomes

Medical
- Assistance may be needed to clear secretions in the setting of a severe respiratory infection.
- The preferred bladder management option is intermittent catheterization for both men and women.
- Self-intermittent catheterization should be learned both in the bed and chair.
- Appropriate bowel management includes a daily or every other day routine on a padded elevated toilet seat.
- Independent for performance of bowel routine with digital stimulation and insertion of suppository or mini enema.
- Typically a digital bowel stimulator or suppository inserter is not needed for bowel routine.

Activities of daily living
- Independent for pressure reliefs using all techniques
- Modified independence with upper body and lower body dressing
- Independent for toothbrushing

- Independent with bathing with adaptive equipment such as a wash mitt, handheld shower, lever type faucet, grab bars, and padded tub bench
- Independent in eating with regular or built up utensils
- Independent with communication and telephoning
- Independent for light meal preparation and light housework
- Assistance needed for heavy housework

Mobility
- Independent driving in a car with modified controls or a van with a captain's seat
- Independent for bed mobility
- Independent with transfers
- Independent with wheelchair propulsion with power or manual wheelchair
- An ultralight wheelchair or power-assist wheelchair is preferred

Vocational
- 8.9% of spinal cord-injured individuals are employed in a professional specialty 15 years postinjury.
- 17% of persons with C5–C8 tetraplegia with a high school diploma are employed.
- Vocational interests do not typically change after an SCI despite an inability to perform activities required for the vocation of interest due to physical limitations.
- 62% of persons with C5–C8 tetraplegia with a master's or doctoral degree are employed.

Participation in sports
- Cycling can be done with an adaptive cycle that allows the participant to use arm cranks to power the cycle.
- The cycle has a third wheel in the front to give it more stability.
- Hand cuffs can be attached to the arm cranks to adapt the cycle for participants who lack strong grasp.
- An abdominal binder can be attached to the participant and the cycle seat to increase trunk stability

Prognosis

Motor recovery
- Most upper extremity recovery occurs during the first 6 months.

- Typically near normal strength and function in the hands can be achieved by 1 year after injury if some T1 motor function is initially present.

Life expectancy

- A 25-year-old can expect to live 36 years, in contrast to the normal life expectancy of 54 years.
- A 50-year-old can expect to live 16 to 20 years, versus normal life expectancy of 31 years.
- A 75-year-old can expect to live 4 to 6 years, versus the normal life expectancy of 12 years.

Helpful Hints

- Rubber bands can be used around the shower handle or soap to make it easier for to grip.

- Side to side or forward lean pressure relief techniques as opposed to push-up techniques should be emphasized in order to limit damage to the shoulders from overuse.

Suggested Readings

Arias E. United States Life Tables 2004. *National Vital Statistics Report.* Dec 2007;59(9).

Consortium for Spinal Cord Medicine. Outcomes following traumatic spinal cord injury: clinical practice guidelines for health-care professionals. *J Spinal Cord Med.* 2000;23(4):289–316.

Fisher CG, Noonan VK, Smith DE, et al. Motor recovery, functional status, and health-related quality of life in patients with complete spinal cord injuries. *Spine.* 2005;30(19):2200–2207.

National Spinal Cord Injury Statistical Center, University of Alabama at Birmingham. *2006 Annual Statistical Report.* July 2006.

Section III: Outcomes

T1 to T9 Paraplegia

Gina Armstrong MD ■ Naomi Betesh DO ■ Thomas N. Bryce MD

Key Innervated Muscles
- All C1–C8 innervated muscles including fully intact upper extremities and diaphragm
- Intercostals
- Erector spinae

Available Muscle Actions
- Some trunk control and stability
- Total control of upper extremities
- Inspiration and expiration

Functional Outcomes

Medical
- Breathing and coughing on own
- The preferred bladder management option is intermittent catheterization for both men and women
- Independent with straight catheterization both in the bed and in the wheelchair
- Appropriate bowel management includes a daily or every other day routine on a padded commode
- Independent performance of bowel routine with digital stimulation and insertion of suppository or mini enema

Activities of daily living
- Independent with pressure reliefs in manual wheelchair
- Independent with feeding, dressing, bathing, grooming, and brushing teeth at the wheelchair level
- Independent with writing and telephoning
- Some assistance needed for heavy housework
- Independent with cooking and light housework such as emptying and loading the dishwasher, doing the laundry, dusting, bed making, and light cleaning
- Front loading washing machines and dryers are ideal for doing laundry at the wheelchair level

Mobility
- Able to stand independently with long leg braces or standing frame
- Not able to ambulate functionally due to energy expenditure needs
- Able to ambulate with long leg braces and walker or crutches for exercise
- Independent for transfers into and out of a car with either a sliding board or popover technique
- Able to drive independently with hand controls
- Independent bed mobility
- Independent for all transfers including floor to chair transfers
- Independent in manual wheelchair propulsion in the community
- Independent in popping a wheelie and ascending and descending curbs

Vocational
- 47% of individuals are working 30 years postinjury.
- 6% of persons with paraplegia and less than a high school education are employed.
- 23% of persons with paraplegia and a high school diploma are employed.
- 70% of persons with paraplegia and a bachelor's degree are employed.
- 75% of persons with paraplegia and a master's or doctoral degree are employed.

Participation in sports
- Wheelchair tennis players must have loss of function of one or both lower extremities.
  - A standard tennis racquet is used.
- Weight lifting competitions for paraplegics include power lifting press and bench pressing.
  - In bench pressing the weight is lifted off a support at chest level.
  - In power lifting the barbell is given to the participant at arm level and the participant lowers it to the chest and then starts the lift from chest level.

Prognosis

Motor recovery
- Only 2% to 3% of persons classified as AIS level A on admission to rehab will progress to AIS level D.
- For persons with complete paraplegia, irrespective of level of injury, lower extremity muscles with grade 1/5 or 2/5 initially can improve to at least a 3/5 over 60% of the time.

Life expectancy
- A 25-year-old can expect to live 41 years, in contrast to the normal life expectancy of 54 years.
- A 50-year-old can expect to live 20 years, in contrast to the normal life expectancy of 31 years.

- A 75-year-old can expect to live 6 years, in contrast to the normal life expectancy of 12 years.

Helpful Hints

- The lower the level of injury, the better the trunk stability.
- Advise persons with decreased sensation never to carry hot items directly on their laps as they are at risk for burns.
- Rolling carts or wooden trays can be used to transport hot food.
- Pants with zippers make it easy for men to straight catheterize.

Suggested Readings

Consortium for Spinal Cord Medicine. Outcomes following traumatic spinal cord injury: clinical practice guidelines for health-care professionals. *J Spinal Cord Med.* 2000;23(4):289–316.

Fisher CG, Noonan VK, Smith DE, et al. Motor recovery, functional status, and health-related quality of life in patients with complete spinal cord injuries. *Spine.* 2005;30(19):2200–2207.

National Spinal Cord Injury Statistical Center, University of Alabama at Birmingham. *2006 Annual Statistical Report.* July 2006.

Waters RL, Adkins R, Yakura J, Sie I. Donald Munro lecture: functional and neurologic recovery following acute SCI. *J Spinal Cord Med.* 1998;21(3):195–199.

T10 to L1 Paraplegia

Gina Armstrong MD ■ Naomi Betesh DO ■ Thomas N. Bryce MD

Key Innervated Muscles
- All C1–T9 innervated muscles
- Intercostals
- External obliques
- Rectus abdominis

Available Muscle Actions
- Neck flexion, extension, rotation
- Trunk flexion/extension/rotation, good trunk control
- Total control of upper extremities

Functional Outcomes

Medical
- The most appropriate bladder management is intermittent catheterization.
- Independent with straight catheterization and applying an external condom catheter if needed
- Appropriate bowel management includes a daily or every other day routine on a commode or padded toilet seat.
- Independent with a bowel routine with manual evacuation of stool if a LMN bowel is present or digital stimulation if an UMN bowel is present

Activities of daily living
- Independent with side-to-side and forward-lean pressure reliefs in manual wheelchair
- Independent with feeding, dressing, bathing, grooming, and brushing teeth at the wheelchair level
- Some assistance needed for heavy housework
- Independent with cooking and light housework such as emptying and loading the dishwasher, doing the laundry, dusting, bed making, and light cleaning
- Front loading washing machines and dryers are ideal for doing laundry at the wheelchair level

Mobility
- Able to stand independently with knee-ankle-foot orthoses (KAFOs) or a standing frame
- Ambulation for exercise may be independent or require some assistance crutches or a walker and KAFOs usually are needed.
- Primary mode of locomotion remains a manual wheelchair.
- Independent for transfers into and out of a car

- Able to drive independently with hand controls
- Independent bed mobility
- Independent for all transfers including floor to chair transfers
- Independent in manual wheelchair propulsion in the community
- Independent in popping a wheelie and ascending curbs
- Independent ascending and descending stairs and escalators in wheelchair

Vocational
- Less than one-third of persons between the ages of 18 and 62 with paraplegia are employed overall.
- Of those with college degrees, almost two-thirds are employed (including 71% of those with a bachelor's degree).

Participation in sports
- Kayaking, canoeing, and rowing can be done with or without adaptations such as outriggers, which make the watercraft more stable in the water.
- Adaptations may also be necessary to make entry and exit from the boats safe for persons with paraplegia.

Prognosis

Motor recovery
- 95% of patients with 1 or 2/5 hip flexor strength at 1 month will recover 3/5 strength in the hip flexors by 1 year.
- Persons with motor complete but sensory incomplete injuries with preserved perianal pin sensation have >75% chance of ambulating at 1 year.

Life expectancy
- A 25-year-old can expect to live 41 years, in contrast to the normal life expectancy of 54 years.
- A 50-year-old can expect to live 20 years, in contrast to the normal life expectancy of 31 years.
- A 75-year-old can expect to live 6 years, in contrast to the normal life expectancy of 12 years.

Helpful Hints
- Advise persons with decreased sensation never to carry hot items directly on their laps as they are at risk for burns.

- Advise the individual to consider changing appliances in the home to a side by side refrigerator/freezer, front loading washer, and dryers.
- Advise the individual to lower counter tops to make them accessible.

Suggested Readings

Apple D. *Physical Fitness: A Guide for Individuals with Spinal Cord Injury.* Baltimore: Department of Veterans Affairs; 1996.

Consortium for Spinal Cord Medicine. Outcomes following traumatic spinal cord injury: clinical practice guidelines for health-care professionals. *J Spinal Cord Med.* 2000;23(4):289–316.

Fisher CG, Noonan VK, Smith DE, et al. Motor recovery, functional status, and health-related quality of life in patients with complete spinal cord injuries. *Spine.* 2005;30(19): 2200–2207.

Krause JS, Kewman D, DeVivo MJ, et al. Employment after spinal cord injury: an analysis of cases from the model spinal cord injury systems. *Arch Phys Med Rehabil.* 1999;80(11):1492–1500.

National Spinal Cord Injury Statistical Center, University of Alabama at Birmingham. *2006 Annual Statistical Report.* July 2006.

Sisto SA, Durin E, Sliwinski MM. *Spinal Cord Injuries Management and Rehabilitation.* 1st ed. Missouri: Mosby; 2009.

L2 to S5 Paraplegia

Gina Armstrong MD ▪ Naomi Betesh DO ▪ Thomas N. Bryce MD

Key Innervated Muscles
- Fully intact arm, abdominal and trunk muscles

Other muscles depend on level of injury
- Hip flexors/abductors/adductors/extensors
- Knee extensors/flexors
- Ankle dorsiflexors/plantar flexors

Available Muscle Actions
- Good trunk control
- Total control of upper extremities
- Partial to full control of lower extremities

Functional Outcomes

Medical
- Appropriate bladder management options for a LMN bladder include Valsalva maneuvers timed with abdominal wall contractions while sitting on a commode or toilet seat or self-intermittent catheterization.
- Independent with straight catheterization, applying external condom catheter and changing urinary drainage bag if needed for males with urinary leakage
- Appropriate bowel management includes a daily morning routine on a padded toilet or commode.
- Independent with bowel routine, which typically includes abdominal massage and inserting finger into rectum to manually evacuate stool

Activities of daily living
- Independent with pressure reliefs
- Independent with feeding, dressing, bathing, grooming. and brushing teeth
- Some assistance potentially needed for heavy housework
- Independent with cooking and light housework

Mobility
- Can stand independently
- Ambulation is functional
- Majority will be community ambulators, although KAFOs or ankle-foot orthoses (AFOs), crutches, or a cane may be needed
- Independent transfers into and out of the car
- Able to drive independently but may need hand controls depending on level of injury

- Independent bed mobility
- Independent for all transfers

Vocational
- 13% of individuals are working 2 years postinjury.
- 16% of spinal cord-injured individuals are students 2 years postinjury.
- 16% of spinal cord–injured individuals work in professional specialties 30 years postinjury.

Participation in sports
- Spinal cord–injured individuals can participate in golf. Automated ball teeing and retrieval aids can be used.

Prognosis

Motor recovery
- Only 2% to 3% of patients classified as AIS level A on admission to rehab will progress to AIS level D.
- For persons with incomplete paraplegia with a neurologic level of injury below T12 who initially have a grade 1/5 or 2/5 hip flexor or knee extensor muscle strength, these muscles can improve to at least grade 3/5, 90% of the time.
- For persons with incomplete paraplegia with a neurologic level of injury below T12 who initially have a grade 0/5 hip flexor or knee extensor muscle strength, these muscles can improve to at least a grade 1/5, two thirds of the time, and to at least a grade 3/5, approximately 20% of the time.

Life expectancy
- A 25-year old can expect to live 48 years, in contrast to the normal life expectancy of 54 years.
- A 50-year old can expect to live 26 years, in contrast to the normal life expectancy of 31 years.
- A 75-year old can expect to live 9 years, in contrast to the normal life expectancy of 12 years.

Helpful Hints
- Community and household ambulators are more likely to have good to normal pelvic control, 3/5 hip flexor strength, and at least 3/5 knee extensor strength in one leg.
- Community and household ambulators are less likely to use bilateral KAFOs.

Suggested Readings

Consortium for Spinal Cord Medicine. Outcomes following traumatic spinal cord injury: clinical practice guidelines for health-care professionals. *J Spinal Cord Med.* 2000;23(4):289–316.

Fisher CG, Noonan VK, Smith DE, et al. Motor recovery, functional status, and health-related quality of life in patients with complete spinal cord injuries. *Spine.* 2005;30(19): 2200–2207.

National Spinal Cord Injury Statistical Center, University of Alabama at Birmingham. *2006 Annual Statistical Report.* July 2006.

Sisto SA, Durin E, Sliwinski MM. *Spinal Cord Injuries Management and Rehabilitation.* 1st ed. Missouri: Mosby; 2009.

Waters RL, Adkins R, Yakura J, Sie I. Donald Munro lecture: functional and neurologic recovery following acute SCI. *J Spinal Cord Med.* 1998;21(3):195–199.

Index